ECHOLALIA

A novel by

Adam Ward Seligman

Echolalia
by *Adam Ward Seligman*

Published by: ☐━○ **Hope Press** P.O.Box 188
Duarte, CA 91009-0188 U.S.A.
SAN 200-3244

Other books on Tourette syndrome by Hope Press:
Tourette Syndrome and Human Behavior
by *David E. Comings, M.D.*
**Ryan – A Mother's Story of Her Hyperactive/Tourette Syndrome
Child** by *Susan Hughes*
Hi, I'm Adam by *Adam Buehrens*
Adam and the Magic Marble by *Adam and Carol Buehrens*
(to order see back leaf)

Library of Congress Cataloging-in-Publication Data

Seligman, Adam Ward, 1961-
    Echolalia : an adult's story of Tourette Syndrome : a novel / by
Adam Ward Seligman.
        p.   cm.
    ISBN 1-878267-31-0 : $11.95
    I. Title.
PS3569.E565E27   1991
813' . 54--dc20
                                                    91-13102
                                                        CIP

Dedication

To Brad Seligman
    who was a source of constant artistic support,

and

Rachel Hambrick
    who served as my muse over most of the first draft.

FOREWORD

A novel is a work of fiction created by the author's vision of the world. As such, certain things remain secrets of the writer's personal symbolism. No one fully expects explanations of why a character has blue eyes or brown - such choices are often arbitrary and artistic. But they are sometimes genetic. In writing this book I came to depend on the comments of a number of readers; friends, doctors, editors, who had certain questions about the medical contents that baffled them. Rather than incorporating them totally into the general text of this novel, which would be dull, I decided a foreword would be more appropriate to explain some of the neuropsychiatric disorders discussed in this novel. I will explain my research into these disorders, and discuss their fictional use.

I have been accused of being autobiographical in my main character Jackson Evans. We both are writers; we both have Tourette Syndrome; we both have had difficulties in interpersonal relationships; we both follow our personal goals and visions. But the differences, especially medical, are many.

i

TOURETTE SYNDROME

Gilles de la Tourette syndrome was first accurately described in 1885 by Dr. Georges Marie Gilles de la Tourette, a student of the great neurologist Charcot at the Salpetriere Institute in Paris. Tourette studied alongside Sigmund Freud and the two were known to have intensely disliked each other. The two differing medical views of Tourette syndrome: psychiatric versus neurological are as much based in their difference of opinion as anything else. Only over the last few years has a truly neuropsychiatric world view of Tourette syndrome emerged.

The importance of this cannot be over-emphasized: It was once thought to be strictly psychological. The pendulum then swung to the opposite extreme and it was thought to be totally biochemical. Now we realize the wonderful diversity of Tourette syndrome as an neuropsychiatric disorder as well as a chemical one. By this realization we free ourselves from both competing world views and a more classical one emerges – a disorder of the brain and also the self, expressed equally by both.

Tourette syndrome is a complex genetic neurological disorder, characterized by chronic multiple tics which wax and wane over time; involuntary vocalizations including sometimes such complicated symptoms as echolalia (repeating others words) and coprolalia (compulsive swearing); and associated disorders which may include in some, but not in all cases, obsessive compulsive disorder (OCD), attention deficit hyperactivity disorder (ADHD), and learning disabilities. Current research indicates an increasing number of behavioral symptoms associated with Tourette syndrome, such as rages, poor impulse control, anxiety, etc.

Whether these are part of the syndrome, or reactions to the social stress of having it, is unclear to me at this time. In Dr. David Comings book *Tourette Syndrome and Human Behavior*, Hope Press, the behavioral and genetic aspects of Tourette syndrome are explored.

My Tourette syndrome symptoms began at the age of seven and a half, while away at summer camp the month after my father died. Memories – so often suppressed – come exploding out of me at times, like Jackson's colors, and my first memory of being different emerges in my memories of the second week of camp. Another boy was sitting on my bunk and when I asked him to move, he made a face at me. I asked him why and he laughed at me. "That's what you do – ALL THE TIME," he responded. My reaction was to land one of the few great punches of my life, directly into his stomach, causing him to run puking to the bathroom. I then noticed that I *did* make faces – eyes blinking, then grimacing, twitches of the neck or shrugs of the shoulder, but what was really worrying me was the fact that my dog Alex had been given away while I was at camp. An irresistible urge to grunt and bark overwhelmed me during this month at camp and sometimes these noises would come out quietly, without my control. I was embarrassed and mortified but could not stop them from occurring. The noises evolved over the next few months, causing the often heralded comment around the Seligman household, "What's the tic of the week?" (The humor inherent in having Tourette syndrome may seem tasteless to some: Without humor, and laughing about your symptoms, psychological survival is almost impossible.)

As I grew older new symptoms would appear and old symptoms would disappear – the classic course of the disorder. When I was nine years old I watched my brother

Echolalia

Brad and my family friend JB playing ping pong. JB missed a shot and swore "Bullshit!". My bark became "bullshit" over the next few days and I was sent home from school frequently for this inappropriate verbal behavior. It was my first emergence of coprolalia, and while it lasted for the next year and half, "bullshit" was the only word. But even that was too much for the public school system I attended. I was diagnosed as psychotic, and expelled from school, starting one of my first fairly serious depressive episodes, which could be another behavioral component of Tourette syndrome. Depression may be a result of the social pressure of having a body out of control, or a related biochemical disorder. Regardless of the cause, it is treatable, and coincidentally some of the strongest drugs used for depression treat Tourette syndrome as well.

I was sent to a special education school in Los Angeles, Park Century, where under the kind supervision of special education instructors I regained my love of learning and discovered how much I liked to read. My first writing comes from this period, but the discovery of *Star Trek* was the crucial step in my development. It led to my first real friend, Matt Asner, and the comradeship of the science fiction world which delights in differences and doesn't discriminate against them. Oh fandom!

Matt and I were frequent visitors at *Star Trek* conventions and while Matt expressed his joy in acting, I became an avid reader of science fiction, and a science fiction writer. When I was fourteen I visited Philadelphia with my eldest brother Joel and on a whim called the editor of *Isaac Asimov's Science Fiction Magazine*, George Scithers. Like many of the great science fiction editors before him – particularly John W. Campbell – he had me over for tea and a conversation about writing for the magazine. The result was my longest story to date, a horribly inaccurate 6,000 word piece about missile defense systems, meteors and a NASA scientist dying of cancer. I was already writing fiction with a biological background, with the chemotherapy and the missile defense system intertwined metaphorically. George rejected it, but complemented me on my characterizations, especially the one of the scientist. I had found my path.

My Tourette syndrome increased and decreased in severity over the next few years; my writing improved for the most part. When I was seventeen I developed coprolalia again, with the words 'cunt', 'fuck', and combinations of the two predominating. These have remained with me the last twelve years. Echolalia showed up as a symptom when I was twenty-six, attending a Tourette Syndrome Association conference in 1987 in Cincinnati. I returned from the conference highly Touretty, and imitating literally every symptom I had seen or heard while there. This continued for several months before burning out of my system like alcohol the day after an all night drunk.

Like Jackson Evans, I was misdiagnosed for a period of time – in my case six years. At the time I was diagnosed, 1976, the average lag between onset of symptoms and correct diagnosis was over ten years. In the succeeding years it has been, through the help of the media, reduced to almost a year, the shortest amount of time possible for a correct diagnosis to emerge. My grandfather, Nathan Bienstock, went eighty years without a correct diagnosis but his symptoms were obvious to the family and he was observed by my neurologist at a Tourette Syndrome Association meeting. After his death his brain was donated to the National Neurological Research Bank, where mine will join him one day, hopefully a long time from now. (But until then I keep the door locked at night in case the researchers get too anxious!)

In Jackson Evans I have created a more complex case of Tourette syndrome than mine, with associated disorders, four in all, combining with his alcoholism, and the psychological problems caused by his twenty years of misdiagnosis. The associated symptoms are not present in all people with this disorder. But they are possible and authors license allows them to co-exist in Jackson Evans.

OBSESSIVE COMPULSIVE DISORDER

Obsessive compulsive disorder is one of the most unusual aspects of Tourette syndrome. It manifests itself as intrusive thoughts which cannot be stopped (obsessions) or actions which cannot be controlled (compulsions). Like Tourette syndrome it has for years been thought to be strictly psychological but like Tourette syndrome its control by medication indicates a strong biological base. In her book *The Boy Who Couldn't Stop Washing*, Dr. Judith Rapoport gives the history of several cases of OCD in moving and compelling personal sagas. Her explanations helped me understand my own obsessive compulsive syndrome which flares up unpredictably under stress, or along with severe Tourette syndrome symptoms. Deciding which symptoms are Tourette syndrome versus OCD is a favorite parlor game of the Tourette syndrome community, and coprolalia seems, in my case, to have a strong basis in OCD, as do many of the more complex ritualistic symptoms.

I didn't know I had OCD until a few years ago when I was discussing some reoccurring thoughts with photographer Lowell Handler, who also has Tourette syndrome. Lowell told me he had similar thoughts and worries and that they were part of OCD. I spoke to my neurologist upon my return and was diagnosed with mild OCD, which in my case took the form of intrusive thoughts of violence or sex. The medications Prozac or Anafranil have helped me at times, as has an understanding that what I was experiencing was a Tourette syndrome symptom rather than a mental problem.

In Jackson Evans, OCD revolves around intrusive literary metaphor; in musical phrases that he can not stop from hearing, and in preoccupations with his Tourette syndrome. Being obsessive about OCD is a classic symptom and very close to my own experience.

SENSORY TOURETTE SYNDROME

In recent years a new wave of thought on Tourette syndrome has been provoked by descriptions of what the patients actually experience while living with Tourette syndrome. A paper published in 1907, *Confessions of a Ticqueur*, the anonymous writings of a Tourette syndrome sufferer, was the first to touch upon this symptom. An article by Tourette syndrome patient Joseph Bliss went into exhaustive detail of the three steps of a Tourette syndrome symptom; the pre-symptom buildup of sensory information, the symptom itself and the post-symptom experience as the brain either decides to tic again or is for the moment satisfied. Dr. Roger Kurlan recently published a paper on sensory Tourette syndrome which looked at the first large population of Tourette syndrome patients who were examined for this aspect of the disorder. Most doctors ignore their patients comments on what they feel around their symptoms. My personal experience, based on discussions with other people with Tourette syndrome, is that sensory Tourette syndrome is quite common in severe cases, less so in milder cases. But whether this reflects greater self awareness of one's own Tourette syndrome or an actual medical phenomenon is unclear at present. In myself I feel a distinct buildup of what I call "pressure" in the center of my body between my diaphragm and throat, sometimes more focused on one than the other. The pressure must be relieved, usually by a vocalization, sometimes by neck jerks. This continues until I have a sense of "doing it right" and the pressure fades away. I associate the color white with this pressure and visualize a column of white air in my body causing some of my symptoms.

SYNESTHESIA

This leads into the most unusual aspect of Jackson Evans' case, the symptoms of synesthesia he feels along with his Tourette Syndrome. Synesthesia can best be described as a cross circuiting of the senses – information which is normally processed by the brain as visual or aural becomes something else. Colors become sounds, taste becomes sensitivity on the skin. The Russian neurologist A.R. Luria studied this disorder in great detail but little is known about it in this country. (In fact, when it is mentioned in our texts, the Russian knowledge is almost always mentioned.)

I first read about synesthesia in a short story by Alfred Bester called *Fondly Fahrenheit* and immediately saw a connection to Tourette syndrome and sensory Tourette syndrome in myself. Other stories which used the theme of brain discharges causing a disorientation of the senses, two in particular by Norman Spinrad (*All the Colors of the Rainbow* and *Carcinoma Angels*) became favorites of mine. It wasn't until I was half way through with the first draft of this book that I found a medical citation linking it to Tourette syndrome. It was, of course, by the wonderful neurologist – writer Oliver Sacks, who in an article makes the comment in a footnote discussing the famous patient of A.R. Luria, about the connection between the *Mnemonist* and Tourette syndrome.

"There are striking resemblances to Tourette's here, not only in the existential conflict between automatism and autonomy (or, as Luria put it, between an 'It' and an 'I'), but in their peculiar and specific neurodynamics, with very rapid, uninhibited, unselective associative neural processes in both - expressed in the *Mnemonist* solely as sensory imagery and synesthesia but in the Touretter, additionally, as 'motor images,' behaviors, enactments or tics."

So in Jackson Evans we have the four disorders, Tourette syndrome, OCD, sensory Tourette syndrome and synesthesia co-existing in a complicated pattern. It enriched me to write about him. While I have checked the medical backgrounds of these neurobehavioral disorders carefully, any mistakes that occur are the result of my imagination and the fictional needs of the novel.

ACKNOWLEDGEMENTS

No novel is written in a vacuum, but this one was an especially well populated island. From the first draft of the first chapter up until publication I relied on friends and colleagues for their opinions and editorial advice.

Many many thanks go to the following people who helped with Echolalia:

Holly Stone, my mother Muriel Seligman, my brothers Brad and Joel Seligman, my sisters and their husbands, Dale Wendel, Lucy Seligman Kanazawa, Don Franzen, Shinjiro Kanazawa, Roxanne Kienly of the Tourette Syndrome Association of Southern California, Jo Anne Clarke, Sue Lynn Levi of the Tourette Syndrome Association, Lynn Sagromosa, playwrite Wendy M. Belden, Rachel Hambrick, Suzanne Madison (hi dolly!) Matt and Ed Asner, Sue Grafton, Jules White, Patricia Oliver Ferguson, Danny Carnahan, Ted Lewis, David Comings M.D., Oliver Sacks M.D., Victoria Ann-Lewis and her writing workshop at the Mark Taper Forum, Randie Rosen, Shelly Stauber Haygood, David Aldridge, Vengoo the Hindoo, Donna Malamud, Jennifer Kirk, Elizabeth Jarvie, Sunshine, William Wharton, Budd Schulberg, Dr. Nadine Payn, Charles Prins, D.C., Amy Freeman, and finally my dog Jaco who ate several pages which needed changes!

I would also like to acknowledge the many works of art by the writers and musicians whose works inspired or consoled me during this project: John Steinbeck, Robert Graves, Robert Silverberg, and musicians Chick Corea, John Patitucci, John Coltrane, John McLaughlin, Peter Erskine, John Scofield (thanks Sco!) Weather Report, Vince Mendoza, Wishful Thinking, Steve Bach, J.S. Bach, Jimi Hendrix, Stravinsky, Matt Zimbel and Manteca, Miles Davis and Sting.

Finally a thank you to my late father Selig Jacob Seligman, whose novel and writings led very directly to my own choice of a career. I wish I had known you better dad.

FOR FURTHER INFORMATION

The Tourette Syndrome Association is an international non-profit health agency devoted to the education of the public and professionals; research funding, and services to people with Tourette syndrome. They have a series of pamphlets and videos for sale as well as an excellent quarterly newsletter for members. I have been a very grateful member for 15 years now, and without them this novel could not have been published for I would not have been diagnosed. To contact them write:

Tourette Syndrome Association
42-40 Bell Boulevard
Bayside NY. 11361
718-224-2999

My audio cassette on Tourette syndrome is now available from Duvall Media, Inc. For a brochure on this and other tapes on Tourette syndrome, write to them at: Duvall Media, Inc. P.O.Box 15892, Newport Beach, CA 92659-5892

Other books about Tourette syndrome, published by Hope Press, are listed on the frontispiece, and can be ordered on the inserted business replay card.

Adam Ward Seligman
Albany, California

ONE

"Sign this one to Linda, okay?"

The man posing the question was dark haired and his black, hostile eyes resembled a panther's, shining and cruel. He was slightly drunk. He had been standing in line for over an hour to get his famous author's signature, served endless amounts of cheap white wine in little clear plastic cups until he was almost angry about finally meeting the writer. The man's hands were soft creased – nails short and bitter – clean but used. They could strangle you as easily as play the piano.

The bookstore was well lit, bookshelves lining the walls and the aisles of book cases well separated for an unsuspecting customer to bend down and reach for a book without getting stepped on by someone on the other side of the corridor of volumes. Music played quietly in the room, gentle stuff, new age music to read books by. Like the light, the corridors, the music was planned out, a trap to lead the reader into the adventure of a lifetime – or dull a long airplane flight.

The writer absorbed this all vaguely from behind the slowly diminishing pile of hard cover books. It was a strange book signing so far, with none of the usual crazies;

instead a manic, nervous crowd that consumed his every word but gave nothing back. The writer signed his name in the book and thought briefly of a line of John Steinbeck's:

"I haven't written because I have been writing."

It felt appropriate to the moment and the writer thought momentarily of saying it out loud. The writer quoted other people constantly in his work, looking for hidden allusions and an underlying structure to fiction. He wanted to share his discoveries. But the dark haired man was gone, off to show Linda his prize, and leaving the writer for an instant in a frightening loneliness – isolation - among the book store crowd. Lonely, lonely lonely, he thought, his eyes blinking out of control for a moment to clear away traces of a slowly forming tear.

"You okay Jackson?"

It was Glenn Otis, the book store owner, greedily gloating over the fifty copies of *Backstabbers!* sold already, and the remaining twenty-five sure to sell by closing. The owner was also a dark haired man and Jackson grimaced – are there no blondes in Hell? he mused to himself, dropping abjectly into his current state of intense self pity. The book he was signing was still on the New York Times best seller list after twenty two weeks, Robert De Niro was set to play the lead character in the motion picture. So what was wrong with this picture? Enough said. Since writing the book three years ago and rewriting (and rewriting and rewriting like the coils of a colossal worm twisting in the mud) the final edit, Jackson Evans hadn't written a word of fiction. Nada. Zero. Nothing created, nothing to follow it up with, no jism of words to delight the screaming masses with. His next planned book was a children's book of light verse, but he saw only dead bodies when he thought of children, little swollen bellies sticking out with milky white powder covering their darkness. He was artistically constipated and felt an internal grief so strong he could barely stand to look at words, his own or even other writers. He hadn't read anything more demanding than People magazine in six months. He hadn't been completely sober in eight. He was destroying himself with his lack of words and an empty creative energy that was exposed best when he was drunk and creating a scene instead of writing one.

"I'm fine, Glenn. I just need to take five, okay?"

The book store owner nodded glumly. He was a dark man inside as well, Jackson noticed unhappily. Glenn thought, this could be the start of the often heralded binge. Gotta keep him away from the white wine.

"Sure Jackson. Take a break. I'll keep the crowd happy."

But not me, Jackson thought despondently. Always please the reader, never the creator. The reader was a wolf, a wolf wearing little old ladies clothes. Clothes? Nightgowns, letters stitched on the sleeves exposing an arm or a milky white thigh. Jackson sighed, thought of the word thigh and felt a momentary excitement. Then it was gone and the dark bellies filled his mind. He looked at a travel book, Africa, and felt the corpses of the famine overwhelming him. He wanted to scream, to cry out in pain as he shut his eyes tightly. Instead he made a sound like a duck quacking and found that satisfied him. The children were gone, replaced by the thought of bare thighs in the sunlight on a beach in the Mediterranean, and he was reminded of Millie pulling on a bathing cap. She laughed at him, and reached out to touch his cheek. He could feel her there, next to him in the book store and he so des-

perately wanted a drink, a Scotch and soda, his father
drank Scotch, his grandfather had been Scottish. As a
child Jackson thought they named the country after the
drink. He opened his eyes and breathed in the room.

A young brunette woman with brown tinted glasses
over her dark shining eyes entered the book store and
zeroed in on Jackson, who was leaning against the wall of
shelves twitching his neck and smoking the pipe that was
his chief affectation. (Actually his name was also an
affectation, but a hidden one. He had been born Jack
Evans: The father begat the child resulting in the addition
of the Son.) The woman surveyed the room and drank in
the loneliness of the crowd. We all want somebody, she
thought. Fools. She walked up to Jackson and said softly,
"Boo!"

Jackson jumped, eyes blinking, and nodded.

"Sara, right, bitch?"

Sara Madison smiled, grateful to be recognized after
last night's first encounter at the publisher's cocktail party
in San Francisco.

"How would you like to be taken out to dinner tonight?"

Jackson thought about it.

"Yeah. I'd like that."

His thoughts leaped around, antelope over the veldt,
then he was back in Africa, the television set showing him
Sally Struthers' well meaning face. He used to get turned
on by Sally Struthers, he thought, then felt the hand of
death pulling at his throat.

The book store owner crept up to them with a fawning
expression.

"Sara! How great to see you again! Keeping an eye
on our star?"

Sara laughed. "He's a big boy. I'm just letting him know that his publisher is buying him dinner tonight. Join us?" Sara asked in a voice that implied nothing could be more distasteful. Glenn shrugged, embarrassed, and muttered something about the wife and kids. Sara pointed at the line of people.

"Get back to work, we have reservations at nine."

Jackson smiled grimly and went back to the long table of books. The owner looked at Sara carefully and said in a low voice with a trace of the intimacy only enemies have for one another, "Is it true that he's six months late with his next book?"

"Well, no ... not exactly."

Sara wanted to hit Glenn, then looked around at Jackson. He was seated again, a patient look on his face hiding none of his pain. Sara wondered what his pain was like. Was it like hers, hidden, still waters and all that? Or was it bigger than life, a grief of the self inflicted kind. Nobody asked you to become famous, she thought. You could have kept your wife. You could still be in debt. But you had to go and write a bestseller. She wondered why she cared and for a angry moment wanted him dead, a moment that was replaced by an even longer one of desire. What the hell was that about? The owner waited for the punchline, breaking Sara's revere.

"But?"

"He hasn't even started it yet. We're a good two years away from another book by Jackson Evans. If he doesn't drink himself to death first."

The alcoholic writers scenario. It was Sara's favorite at college.

"He's got to stop swearing at the customers. I had to refund one woman earlier today because he called her a

5

'bitch.' "

"That goes with the territory. He has some nervous condition that gets worse under stress."

"Fuck stress. If he upsets another person, I will demand your house pay for the refund."

Sara lit a cigarette and let the smoke blow softly into Glenn's face.

"We paid for the wine. I'll be here until closing. Don't worry."

The owner went back to the book signing table, grabbing a fried shrimp from one of the caterers on the way. It was slightly greasy and Glenn gagged for a second. Food was almost as important as sales, almost, but not quite.

"Sign this one to Patricia, with love Jackson."

Jackson put his pen down slowly and looked the young tee shirted woman in the eye. She was about twenty- two, thin, athletic. She wasn't blonde but had long hair down to her waist. Jackson wanted to fuck her. He was swelled with a blind desire from the one eyed demon.

"I have a better idea, let's check into a hotel room and I'll give you an autograph you'll never forget."

Laughter, polite, refined but teetering on hysteria.

"Pardon me?"

"No, pardon me. You want my love, you'll have to prove it. One signature, one roll in the hay, bitch ... "

The crowd erupts outward from the table, grumbling, Jackson the bitter focus once again. Glenn grabbed Jackson tightly and shoved him against a wall. "Are you out of your mind? This kind of behavior is very unprofessional."

"This fucking room is so wrapped up in ink stains that they don't see, don't listen. She'll forget it in five min-

6

utes." Jackson chuckled.

"I already have. Miss ... ?"

Reaching for a cup of wine, Jackson Evans swoons slightly, crashing into a display of Robert Heinlein's last book. The stand falls over, dead, sliding paperbacks across the floor like the corpse of Heinlein. Glenn motions to Sara and turns to the now emptying book store and the man on the floor.

"You fucking drunk, we have another ten copies we could have sold. Don't you care about your career?"

Sara walked up quickly and helped Jackson to his feet. He staggered for a moment, neck twitching wildly, and grunts emerging from his throat like a wild animals. People stopped to stare, then would hurry outside then came back inside to see the rest of the show. It was a circus with one ring, or rather, a noose.

"I have no career. Miss ... ?" Jackson said.

Glenn waved his hand as if brushing at flies.

"No more to drink, damn it! You have another twenty minutes of signing to finish, then you can get the hell out of my store."

Jackson nodded agreeably. Empty book store, empty hotel room, empty heart. Dinner would be a nice distraction, a pretty woman - although not blonde - and a bottle of the red as Papa Hemingway would have said. Jackson reached for his pen, and stared obsessively at a blotch on his right thumb. Ink stain. Semen from the pen's core. Semen was on his mind lately. That and death. Death from starvation, death from lack of sex. The internal ache inside needing to be dulled again from the cup. He wanted a Scotch so badly that he could almost taste it, ashes in his mouth from his pipe, ashes ashes, the black death born again breathed out from his mouth and absorbed an entire room. Morbid bastard, he wanted to shout. Can't you control anything, your mind, your life? What was so important about starvation to you, you're going to dinner silly fool, dinner, and then back to the image of the baby's corpse.

Sara stood behind him, delight showing as he signed the last copy of his novel. Jackson stretched, and looked at the last three disappointed people in line.

"We're out, so scat!"

Glenn cringed and talked quietly to the three customers, calming them down. "He's been under a lot of strain lately, and has had too much to drink ... "

People were always apologizing for his behavior. From the age of twelve to the age of thirty-five. Treating him like a God damned child or an idiot in an institution. What if he apologized? Dare he disturb the structure of his universe? I grow old, he thought sadly, wishing for the mermaids to come. The sea and Eliot. Good old Thomas, he thought, then realized that he too was dead. Was the whole world dead? It was Eliot who said it ended not with a bang but a whimper. More like a whinny, and he started to make horse noises out loud. Glenn looked at him, startled, and Jackson grabbed onto Sara's arm nervously.

Sara patted his twitching neck and smiled. "No permanent damage to your reputation I hope. Do you like Persian food?"

"Shish kabob, that sort of thing?"

They impaled people, that's what they said in the history books. But was it Persia, or modern day Iran where they did that? It was close, he thought. Iran is close to Africa, and the images blotted out his brain again, flies now crawling over the corpses and Jackson finding pleasure that at least, the flies were alive. For the moment anyway.

"Yes. Shish kabob."

"Love it. Reminds me of 'Kubla Khan' ... that wasn't finished either, was it now?"

"Pardon?"

Jackson shrugged. "Never mind. Just a poem ...writers block, visitor... "

Sara looked concerned then grabbed his hand in hers. "Let's go."

And away they went.

TWO

The restaurant on Solano Avenue didn't seem to be Persian: It was more like Yuppified California Cuisine in style and presentation. Watercolored prints of California seashore scenes decorated the walls while the waiters wore blue jeans and red fezzes. But the food was good, the wine was good, the company ...

Sara was saying brightly, " ... Any thoughts on your next book Jack?"

She was calling him Jack already. Usually women didn't take liberties with his pen name. It was a security, say the name own the man. But ownership of a name was one thing, of a man another. Sara wanted to take back the name, to call him Jackson instead or even Mr. Evans. But it was too late, the intimacy had been broached and he turned a weary bloodshot eye on her and she felt a tingle inside. He looked like Hell. Good. Jackson considered this. He could lie, yet again, and say that he was hot on his next potentially best selling book. Or he could tell the truth, something he avoided at the best of times; particularly around women. His wife had believed his lies, up until a point, but after fifteen years of wedded bliss had crawled into bed with his best friend. Since then, well since the divorce, he had had no women in his life and few friends. Life seemed safer that way.

"You know, bitch, I have this nervous disorder."

Jack leaned under the table and pulled off his sandals. He was submerged a long time and Sara nervously crossed her legs. Jackson came up holding a fork, the tines bent almost in half.

"I had noticed." Sara curled her forehead in thought, crinkling her nose underneath her eyeglasses. Jackson found it delightful.

"What's it called again?"

"Tourette syndrome. I always felt it was something that only travel agents could get."

Sara laughed politely at his witticism, then studied Jackson slowly. His sandy hair was receding slightly, his eyes dancing colors in the candle light. She wondered if one eye was different in color from the other. "What's your point?"

"I want to write about it."

Jackson paused and savored the word. Write. It was a simple word, one syllable, rhyming with the word right. As in all right. Jackson realized he was obsessing on the word and pulled himself back to the dinner.

"The doctors tell me I have a very mild case, some facial tics, racing thoughts. I want to look at Tourette syndrome from a novelist's viewpoint, write a book about it that in some way explains it and ... "

Jackson's words dribbled off, and he began staring

10

down intently at the table, suddenly embarrassed for some reason as though he were naked among strangers. Something about Sara made him very uncomfortable and he was slow to realize it was the fact that she was comfortable with him, an odd occurrence in his life. Most people, hell, most women were so put off by his outbursts, his tics, that they built up walls of glass between themselves and him. Jackson would sometimes try to scale these walls only to break through to find himself uninvited in a house of mirrors with no one inside.

"And what?" Sara pushed, curious.

He had walked into that question.

"Helps. Myself, others in my life. You know," Jackson said quickly, changing the topic, "I drink too much."

Sara smiled. "I had noticed."

Yes, she had. It was part of the fascination that Jackson had for her. Daddy had drunk too much, but had gone far without the additional handicap that Jackson was facing. These days it seemed everybody did something too much, drank, smoked, fucked, whatever. Except Sara who kept to her room and waited for her prince to ride in on a white stallion. Jackson continued,

"I think it's to compensate for what I feel building up inside me, pent up rage, more extreme tics, louder noises."

Sara leaned back onto the pillow by the tableside.

"You're thinking out loud. It's nice Jack. You haven't thought as a writer in a long time. Will this be like *Backstabbers!* or more like your first book?"

Jackson looked away from Sara, embarrassed again. My God! he thought to himself, I'm attracted to her! There was a controlled energy to her, a steadiness of purpose that reminded him of Millie before she got all hard edged. At the same time Sara had a little girl quality, a barely

11

concealed vulnerability that made Jackson relaxed. He could dominate her, not be overwhelmed by her the way Millie had overwhelmed him at first. Jackson was starting to get excited by her interest. My God, he thought, I could actually start writing again!

"I think it could transform my writing from contemporary fiction to literature."

"That's all to the good," Sara commented in her best business voice, "but would it sell?"

A stab but a good one. Jackson had winced.

"Fucking editorial assistant. The bottom line, the red versus the black, drowning in gas ..."

Jackson stopped and chuckled. He looked at her very directly, and she raised her glasses back over her eyes nervously.

"This book could really be very sexy."

He looked at Sara very intently, waiting for her to look away. She finally matched his stare, then she reached under the table for his foot and stroked it in a soft warm dry hand. He had a callous under his big toe and she wondered nervously if his feet were clean. Where were his socks?

"I'm involved, Jack ..." Sara lied. She lied well, having been trained by the best in the publishing business. But she almost didn't want to lie to Jackson. She wanted to feel his arms around her ... what was she thinking? That was dirty, you get diseases that way and it could lead to something she couldn't handle, like a relationship. Put him off, box him in, but don't join him, ever. Sara laughed and moved her hand cautiously to Jackson's thigh - he let it rest there, sensing her involvement was with him, at least for the moment. Could he keep her attention? That would be the test.

"Your movements, what do you call them? Tics?" Sara asked.

"Or twitches. Riches bitches." Jackson laughed, and Sara laughed with him.

"The noises, are they also tics?"

"You could call them verbal tics. They feel the same."

Sara blinked. "You're aware of them then? You seem so unaffected by them."

"I don't consciously pay much attention to them but the discomfort if I don't tic is worse than if I do."

"What does it feel like? An itch?" Sara didn't know where her interrogation was taking her but she felt she was onto something, a clue to his sadness.

"What do the tics feel like? You know how when you walk along the beach and you see a seashell you can almost hear it before you pick it up? You know the sound a butterfly in the distance makes as its wings scrape together? It feels like that, a tingle but not a tingle, a pain that doesn't hurt but cuts right into your being like a sharp knife into butter. I tingle. If I wanted to right now I could knock this table over and scream and kick. But I don't. I suppress those extreme movements and sounds, and instead bitch I bitch shit instead I swear."

Sara held his foot tightly, feeling the muscles tense then relax in her hand.

"Such control," she whispered. "It must be hard."

"If you keep on tickling me it will be," Jackson said with a leer. Sara stopped, embarrassed, and the two of them looked away from each other, the moment fading into the next. The waiter hovered - a black cloud in a red fez on the meals horizon.

"Will there be anything else tonight?"

Jackson looked at Sara. "Cognac?"

13

She nodded, knowing it would prolong what must not be, but felt right at the moment.

"Two cognacs."

The waiter smiled darkly then strode away. Jackson moved his foot so her hand was higher up his thigh, closer to his crotch. Sara pulled back but he reached for her hand and held it a moment.

"It's very lonely being a writer," he began, "an occupation best kept in solitude."

Sara squeezed his hand a moment then pulled her hand away.

"Please don't Jack. I'm not in the mood for a pass right now. Maybe we should go ... "

"This is my home town, you know." Jackson said, changing the subject yet again.

"Berkeley?"

"Albany actually ... "

"I thought you were from Los Angeles?"

"I just worked there for the last eight years. I moved there right before my parents died."

"I'm sorry," Sara said simply.

Jackson continued, ignoring her words for the moment but letting them register in the receptors of his mind.

"Here I can try to relax and try to remember. Things spinning out of control, the falcon cannot hear the falconer ... "

"Keats right?" Sara said, trying to impress him. (English had been her one weak point at Vassar.)

"Actually Yeats, but Keats had his moments too. The Eve of St. Agnes rests somewhere inside me, burdening my soul with its wintry message."

Sara moved her hand back to Jackson's leg. He held it, then looked at his watch.

14

"What time is the flight to Los Angeles tomorrow?"

"Afternoon, threeish, I think."

"Feel like some music? Dancing, listening, blues clubs?"

Sara smiled. It would take some of the pressure off, postpone making a commitment to Jackson, even if just for the night. Sara hated commitment, yet did everything in her power to find it. Jackson seemed after something else - sex, or something more pristine like love. Oh, fuck it, she thought. He's just horny.

"I'd love to hear some music."

"We can observe, the novelists favorite preoccupation!"

Jackson rat-a-tatted a rhythm on the table loudly. Sara jumped then grinned.

"Or maybe I'll sit in."

Sara was finding herself more and more intrigued by Jackson. It could just be the brandy she thought. But his self pity, combined with his wit and his genuine loneliness touched her in some way. He reminded her of someone - herself perhaps, before therapy, and EST. But they had ultimately failed and she realized that true happiness revolved around a regular paycheck and a safe apartment building without the fear of assault.

"When you write ... " Sara started, then stopped, worried that it would seem like a criticism. At this moment she didn't want to be too critical of Jackson.

"When I write, which isn't often these days. Go ahead Sara, ask your questions, I've heard them all before."

Oh no, he sounds bored.

"What I meant was, do you need to drink as much, does writing give you the same kind of high?"

"That question wasn't the one I expected. Yes and no.

15

I drink to unwind and you have no idea how a best selling book increases your tension level. I was not made for fame – I just want to put words together into sentences that evolve into books. That's all."

"Bullshit! You must be after more than that. You have so much passion in you – in your eyes, in your voice ... what am I saying?"

"Yes, hopefully."

"Let's go hear some blues. I want to hear you drum on a real drum set."

"That would be a good start."

And away they went.

THREE

Sara Madison hadn't always been a editorial flack for a publishing house, but it was her first 'legitimate' job. As she tells it, she blundered into it, just like she blundered into being an "A" student at Vassar, a part time actress off Broadway, and finally a researcher for a national sports magazine. At the time she and Jackson Evans were listening to the beautiful bowed bass playing of Eddie Gomez at Yoshi's, she had successfully avoided any hint of a relationship lasting more than three weeks. At twenty-five she was tuned tightly twined like Gomez' bass, her heart resonating off her mind and creating a blurred perspective from which all men were basically pigs or father figures. Now hear her song, in three quarter time, metronome set at 90 beats per minute.

> I that loved,
> loved little,
> that I loved,
> loved less.

> I wander,
> confused, yet hesitant
> about the state of my
> confusion.

> When I go,
> I move,
> fast slow,
> pass go,
> then wither quietly,
> in a man's arms.

> Beside me sits the writer,
> inside me sits the reader,
> the perfect couple,
> the imperfect reality of
> lives lived learning,
> Yearning for release,
> but too scared to ask,
> to demand,
> to beg,
> or just to be.

FOUR

At the age of twelve strange things start to happen to people. The racing hormonal lurch that we all enter into throws you for a loop, a spin, and sometimes sets you up for a fall. When Jack was twelve he began to see voices, to hear visions, to taste colors – red red red as death – to breathe water, to fly on wings of cold steel. He blinked often, and his neck would jerk out of control at times when he was excited. His family was bewildered.

MOTHER: It's just a stage.
FATHER: A stage in what show?
MOTHER: The play's the thing, wherein we'll find ...
FATHER: ... And speak of many things ...

Voices in the wind outside the Albany schoolyard, shooting up to Kensington where the rich folk lived, floating over the East Bay grief stricken and laughing. What is wrong with me? Jack would ask himself, then retreat into strange fantasy worlds of mermaids and vampires, searching for him in the deep water, or just skulking around his bedroom window at night. He began to keep a journal ...

JANUARY – I heard them again this morning,
plotting. They saw me again last
night, spotting.

FEBRUARY – Are they real?
Should I squeal?

MARCH – In like a lying,
Out on the lam ...

Others were aware of his preoccupation. At school they made extensive notes in his permanent record, which would haunt him throughout his high school years. "Dreamy, out of touch, easily distracted," ran one of the entries. "Prone to being here but ditching mentally," ran another. Even Mister Barker, whom Jack liked for his dry wit and command of English, would in later years write, when receiving Jackson's novel *Lucia*, "that Evans as a child had a rare command of his fantasy life. But I wouldn't want to have to share it with him. The book is dark, like Jack as a boy, Jackson as a man."

APRIL – Come the Showers,
Lose the powers.

MAY – Jack be nimble, Jack be quick,
God almighty I must be sick!

JUNE – Even the birth of summer
Seems to make me dumber.

The rock fight lasted a day and a night, neighboring kids tossing pebbles, then rocks, at each other up and down the street, breaking windows in the process. It was a teenage ritual, a taking of manhood with all of memories of the hunt for wild game and the chase for position within the teenage tribe on this street. Jack went out at first to watch, then to observe, then finally to join in the mayhem. He stood on the balcony of his two story home, tossing mud clots down on the more aggressive throwers who ran with Millie Benjamin until he became not just a participant but THE ENEMY.

"School's out!" became the rally cry that they all threw the rocks to. When the injuries started – bruises, cuts, abrasions – there was laughter, warm sweaty guffawing. When Jack was struck hard in the head with a rock, knocking him to the ground and splitting his lip, red red red blood pouring out of him like dwarf stars against the milky way, the laughter stopped and the frightened but proud rock throwers ran home.

Jack started to blink a lot more after that and sometimes his thoughts raced even faster than before, words and voices and colors – red red red – fastening him into a dark depression. Did it trigger his later problems or were they always there hidden by his humor and boyish energy? No one seemed to know.

JULY –   I feel the heat in my eyes,
                    Yet fear the broken sties.
AUGUST –   No matter what they do or say,
                    I won't escape them anyway.
SEPTEMBER – Bells again in the schoolyard,
                    Flags at half mast in the shipyard.

In September Jack Evans was diagnosed as psychotic, living in a dream world where all colors hinted at a taste or a sound. His parents visited various residential homes but decided to treat Jack at home, a tutor appearing every day from school for a couple of hours to relieve mother and father from the chore of keeping Jack away from sharp objects – pointed things – wires and the eternal urge to smash the hi - fi.

The soundtrack for Jack's condition was relentless as the Beatles faded into the hard rock of Led Zeppelin, classical piano, the sound of waves upon an empty beach - can one hear that which is unheard? Jack wondered - the drive of pulsing groove giants like the Brecker Brothers floating into a Rolling Stones revival and always in the background a radio hum buzzing BUZZ in Jack's ears.

OCTOBER –   Pay the rent daddy-OH
            Life is spent Mommy-OH
NOVEMBER – In the sweet darkness I will lie,
            In the cold moonlight I will die.
DECEMBER – The death of another year
            Fills me with unspoken fear

In the end it all turned out to be a concussion that was proceeded by the tortured visions of red red red and the sound the surf makes in the silvery moonlight.

Sure. Tell me another one.

Okay – Jack was crazy. He was nuts – gaga – mental. But did that explain the tics, the strange sensations he described to the unhearing psychiatrists with their ready-made diagnosis for what they could not understand? No it didn't. When Jack began to curse they said he was becoming violent, that he would have to be institutionalized definitely now for his parents safety. But his parents only saw a frightened little boy and when Jack peered into his bathroom mirror and saw his fourteen year old face so old, so young, he was haunted by the red red red tint that covered it.

FIVE

It was a week later, another smog filled city, another dingy first class hotel room, on this endless spring book promotion tour which had lasted for three weeks now and had another two weeks to go.

"No Jack," she said, kissing him one last time, savoring his taste on her lips. How had they ended up on his bed?

Jackson pulled away from Sara's arms and stared at her intently. "No?" He asked.

"No. I don't do this."

Jackson sat up, lit his pipe and watched the smoke curl to the ceiling of his hotel room. He took his shoes off, and curled his toes until they cracked. Sara jumped at the noise. "You know, Sara, I like you. I like you a lot. I like you more than ... it's been long time since I felt comfortable with anyone. But we're going to be on the road together for another two weeks and this could simplify things for both of us ... "

"Or complicate them."

"Jesus!" Jackson leaped to his feet, pulling off his green and white striped sweater, and going to the window. "It's all out there, you know, in this city. Nobody else sees it or feels it but I can hear the storm clouds forming." Storm clouds with a silvery lining.

"What?" Sara asked, buttoning up her blouse, and wondering if she had pushed him away for good. Damn it, I have to stop being so scared!

"What are you raving about now Jack?" She asked,

laughing at the intimacy of his first name nervously.

"My book."

"*Backstabbers!?*"

"No, the new one. I decided at dinner tonight, after the shellfish actually, where was I? Oh yes, to try writing again, but now I just wonder if it would be empty like you and me, or more impassioned, like the never ending song in my head ... "

Sara lay back again on the bed, her eyes questioning but unimpressed by what she perceived as Jackson's latest strategy to get into her skirt. "I think I'll let you work this one out by yourself Jack." His hand on her breast had been so warm with odd callouses from years of playing drum set. She wanted to rock in rhythm underneath them, then laughed inside at her cliched mind.

"I could request you, as my liaison with Rockford House. You'd like that, wouldn't you, the opportunity to work closely with me on my next book, you would, wouldn't you?"

Sara smiled and motioned to Evans to come closer. "All this just to get me into your bed, or is this real life, Jack? Will you write another book? Chances are you're a one trick pony, well two, if you count the opera one ... "

"Lucia?" Jackson asked, nodding his head. "I do count that. It was a much tidier book to write – no fame and reviewers hanging over my fingers waiting for the nails to be clipped into a prose style, which then they could declare was the Jackson Evans style, indistinguishable from the style of any other writer the critics pretend to understand. But they can't understand me, I don't understand me, and I live me twenty-four hours a day. How can you have a style after just one book? Hemingway did but Steinbeck didn't find one for years and Fitzgerald was so lost in the bottle that what little style he had was wasted away, snow melting over sterile rocks ... "

Jackson sat on the edge of the bed and Sara touched the back of his head gently. His neck twitched and he felt for her hand but it slipped away into the night as she stood up. "Good night Jack. I'll see you in the morning."

"Night Sara." Jackson considered for a moment. "I need a drink if you're going."

Sara felt like an accomplice to Jack's addiction. "You shouldn't drink anymore Jack. You've had enough."

"Then stay and hold me."

Sara moved closer to Evans then suddenly stopped. "I'll call room service for you then. Scotch?" God I'm such a bitch sometimes, but he's too exposed right now, too emotionally naked.

"Bitch."

"Just doing my job."

"In that case make it brandy."

Sara swore and left the hotel room. Jack saw red red red for a moment in the rustle of her skirt, then lay back. What do I really know about? Voices colors images sentences ... all linked together in my never stopping brain waves and neural firings. He sat up and wondered if he had a legal pad with him ...

Into the night he sketched and pondered a world in which someone like him lived, a man with all of his physical problems but none of the spiritual defects he saw in himself. A man whose emotions and desires were naked to the world and was an example with his honesty. Who was it that was honest? George Washington was said to be honest but he was also a man of war. Gandhi was a living saint but maybe too saintly and there were the young girls he slept with. No, go back, farther back into history, look

24

for him, got it! Diogenes looking with that lantern for the honest man or was it the honest landlord ... Christ, I better turn in now, it's getting late. Christ ... He was honest too. What a story that would make, the son of God reborn in today's world, today's ... Jackson sat up and grinned. Got it!

SIX

He knows when she's right,
Yet he wants to fight,
Not give up when hope is in sight.

Desire is a heady beast,
That grows like so much yeast,
And flows West to East.

Desire is a heady brew,
It is a stage cue,
From the mind regarding what to do.

I want her, he thinks.
I want her, he says and takes a drink
From a cup half filled with beer.

I want her he cries,
I want her he sighs,

25

Echolalia

And then he calls her dear.

He understands (Or so he tells her)
He understands he wants her
To come Westering with him,
To Pacific Ocean swim
And be with him
In the deep – the blue blue deep.

She understands her feelings,
That leave her reeling,
With a sticky sweat on her thighs -
A stunned look in her eyes,
Like a fallen deer facing the
Shotgun blasts of passion.

She understands but wants not to hurt him,
Not knowing that in the ocean swim,
Many whims,
And desires,
And fancies that trickle down one's legs,
To one's feet
And causes one to beg,
And sometimes to plead.

But desire is not to be tamed,
Or caged,
Or caught,
But only held taut,
In one's minds eye,
So you can buy time,
Until you're ready,
To drink from the cup of desire.

Airline tickets are cheap,
But hearts are not,
My dear.
When you're ready you'll reap
The heady grapes that are caught
In my cup of beer.

Until then I have you in my head,
Wishing you were in my bed,
But understanding,
Oh too well,
That some things had to be said,
About desire.

SEVEN

"Dr. Collins will see you now Mr. Evans." Nurse Smith said. Jackson smiled at the nurse and wondered why she seemed not to notice his eyes blink blink blinking out of control. He wanted to ask her about this, why she didn't seem to notice, but instead he felt an urge to shout 'bitch' at her. These urges had been increasing for months now until they totally consumed him. Last month he had seen a neurologist about it after his general practitioner diagnosed a seizure disorder. He had gone for test after test, PET, MRI, CAT, EEG, all of it just so much alphabet soup to him. Now the specialist, the neuropsychiatrist for God's sake (whatever that was,) will explain to me that I'm just plain insane and should be locked up for my good. Won't that just delight Millie, the bitch! He held his hands tightly together for a moment, stroking the inner palm of his right one, then his left.

Dr. Timothy Collins was a thin man, almost like a cadaver, thought Jackson. He was pale, with sandy white hair and sky blue eyes. He wore a white jacket with his name embroidered lightly in blue by his wife Betty upon it. It fit him tightly as though it had been a size too small at one point. He nodded kindly at Jackson and said cheerfully, "I read your book last night. Very good."

"Thank you. I wish the critics had been as nice."

Dr. Collins laughed, not sure if it were a joke or not. "Mr. Evans, I have some good news for you and some bad. You don't have any kind of brain tumor according to the CAT scan that Dr. Brady ordered. You have no progressive disease ... "

Jackson twitched his neck and stared intently at Dr. Collins, almost daring him to comment on it. "That leaves mental, right? I'm going insane. Again."

"Not at all, even considering your possible misdiagnosis as a child."

"Misdiagnosis? I was considered psychotic for four years. They were wrong about that?"

"Doctors are often wrong about this disorder. It is classically misdiagnosed."

Jackson's heart double timed for a moment then he sighed in resignation. "What disorder?"

"Mr. Evans, have you ever heard of Tourette syndrome?"

"No." Oh God, not another name - another label for my quirks! Does the labeling ever end? "Is that what I have?"

28

"Yes. And no. Your case is kind of unusual, with the things you describe. I think you have what is beginning to be called sensory Tourette syndrome. You have a preponderance of images which come out brilliantly controlled, as in your writing, or uncontrolled as in your tics, racing thoughts, coprolalia ... "

Jackson interrupted. "Copro what?"

"Involuntary swearing. About a third of the patients we see have this symptom. It's a classic sign of the disorder, although Gilles de la Tourette thought echolalia was the dominant symptom."

"Echolalia." The word echoed rapidly through Jackson's mind and he felt almost a giddiness. Not insane! Not to die! "What a beautiful word. You say I have that too?"

"You have a tendency towards reoccurring thoughts, that could be described as mental echolalia or OCD, which you also exhibit."

"Whoa." The giddiness stopped. "Stop throwing terms at me and tell me when I'm going to die."

"You're not, at least not from Tourette syndrome. Your drinking may kill you, your history indicates that you're very addictive at times, when you're not creating. But Tourette syndrome in of itself is not fatal. There are some medications you could take but I think your case is too mild to warrant them. I think if you could avoid stressors, caffeine, alcohol, exercise more, maybe see a psycho-therapist to work through some of your anger ... "

"Uh. Okay." Jackson stopped him and the room spun for a moment. He saw the earth, dry rotting with drought and he knew that it wasn't over yet. "So I got this thing I've never heard of but it won't kill me. Is that it?" Lord does it ever end? When will I be normal, just like the rest of the confused people I meet at work, or in the nightclubs who only want to get laid perfectly in a normal non neurotic way. I just want to be like them but not to lose my gift, my writing. Is there a middle ground, will the center ever hold?

"The rest depends on you Mr. Evans. There's a Tourette syndrome support group that meets every month in Los Angeles. You could try going to it, compare experiences, lose some of that mantel of self pity which you wear so well ... "

"Pardon me, Dr. Collins, it's not self pity but writers block. Do you have any idea of what it's like to lose a major part of yourself, to be wordless, impotent with paper etched white with grief ... "

Jackson was getting angry by Dr. Collins insensitivity or what he perceived as insensitivity. Actually Dr. Collins found Jackson fascinating but his celebrity status made Dr. Collins shy around him. *Backstabbers!* had come out to rave reviews and the thought that he had a famous patient with Tourette syndrome instead of the typical waiter or unemployed student with multiple tics frightened Dr. Collins. What if he were wrong in his diagnosis, would Jackson sue? Malpractice was like a greedy vulture at Prometheus' liver these days.

Dr. Collins looked at Jackson closely, then shook his head.

"No, it's still self pity. Give up drinking, coffee, and unwind a little. Go see a basketball game, laugh, mastur-bate, whatever it takes to become fully human again, because you're failing at it now, that I can assure you." Lord that was blunt!

Jackson smiled. "Yeah, I don't like you very much either Doc." He rose to go. "But when I get in touch with this thing, this Tourette syndrome, watch out. Because then

I'm going to flame out in glory."

Dr. Collins nodded and shook hands with Jackson. "Good luck finding it."

Jackson went to the Hamburger Hamlet on Van Nuys Boulevard and drank an Irish Coffee while eating their tiny onion rings and a cheeseburger named after Rex Harrison. He looked at the articles Dr. Collins had given him on Tourette syndrome and decided that it made sense as a diagnosis. It would be nice to be able to call his parents and tell them he wasn't crazy, but their death in a car accident shortly after *Lucia* came out made it impossible. So he called Millie.

Millie was strangely delighted by the news and wanted to have dinner and talk about her alimony checks. She too had seen the reviews of *Backstabbers!* and was happy with them, but for different reasons. Jackson made a dinner date, thought about ripping off her breasts and wondered how come Dr. Collins didn't reassure him about the thoughts being so violent at times. He wanted to hurt Millie, but he also felt some strong sexual feelings for her as well. He knew that their relationship was the only one he had ever had and despite the way the divorce had gone, she was his first and only lover. She had believed in him, still did in fact. Why then the urge to hurt her? He wanted to call Dr. Collins back and ask him and started to dial the number. He stopped. That could wait for his next appointment, the week before the book signing tour with Rockford House. For now he wanted another drink and then it was time to go back to work at Dig It! Two more days, he thought to himself, then I stop my day job and can go on with my life, my writing.

If only I had something to write about, something unique to say. It was that fear more than anything else which stopped Jackson from writing now. What if he was just a hack?

What if he were? Hacks have to eat too, you know. Besides, even Faulkner wrote for Hollywood.

EIGHT

Millie Benjamin was fascinated by Jack Evans. Although six months younger then he was, at fourteen, she was infinitely wiser in the ways of the world, having been turned on to sex, drugs and rock and roll at age thirteen by the neighborhood rock throwers. She used to walk home with Jack, watching him exploding inside after school with noises and twitches and speaking of the 'voices' he was hearing in his head all the time now. She knew he wasn't nuts, just weird, but when he stopped going to school because of his diagnosis of psychosis, she defied her father's orders to be with him in the late afternoons, staring across the street to the Albany bayside race track, wondering if their phantom bets would ever land any real money.

Millie was still quiet, stuck inside her head with fantasies about her future. She wanted to be a singer, not interested in being a rock star like her friends but a Maria Callas born again. She would practice arias in the shower each morning and her father, Saul, would take her into the city to hear the San Francisco Opera Company during the season. Her favorite operas were the extravagant ones, big stories with big characters. Her initial attraction to Jack was in the fact that he was a story teller; a creator. But there was a physical side to it too, a desire for his arms around her.

Millie wondered what Jack would be like as a lover but never dared push his hormonal buttons for fear that he would freak out on her and reject her. Jack wondered what she felt like, tasted like, looked like for God's sake if he – she – it actually existed. So the two of them grew frustrated together and talked of many things, all true to their age and to Jack's strangeness.

"I sometimes feel like I'm going to explode one day, just turn red red red inside and never come down." Jack would say, his neck twitching in rhythm with his internal music.

Millie would put her tan and freckled hand on his shoulder and ask what he meant by red red red. "You use that term so much but it seems so unclear to me. What do you see, the color behind your eyes when you shut them?"

Jack would try to explain, his horniness distracting him but Millie's genuine interest exciting him. "It's like there is this whole different world inside me, of colors bursting into song, of tastes melting into voices, of sounds hitting me on the face and slapping me into screaming 'yes it's me I'm alive!' It seems like there's always music in my head, loud rhythmic, intense. But the music isn't exactly a tune I know or ever heard. I want to correct it, play all the notes right but after awhile it becomes a blur, a cacophony of noise. When I play drums I try to play to that music."

"You're a great drummer Jack. Maybe that inner music makes you special in some way, unique."

Jack smiled at Millie. "But I don't know how it's

different from what you see and feel. I know you don't feel the red red red lapping against your brain, you say you don't anyway. I just wonder ... "

"Wonder what, Jack?" Millie asked excited by the conversation, the sheer intimacy of it all, the strangeness of Jack's mind.

"If I'm really going mad. Maybe I am crazy. Maybe you shouldn't be here with me."

"Why not," Millie asked, her chest touching Jack's arm. He could feel her taut nipple against his skin through her tee shirt and he felt a building up of rage red red red that she was teasing him even as she felt his lack of interest as an insult. So it went, the eternal dance between them.

"I want to do things with you sometimes Millie, and I know we shouldn't but I see the two of us alone all this time and feel constrained to ... to touch you."

"You can touch me Jack. Please touch me." Millie felt relieved that her need was out and wondered if Jack would respond to it in a way she would like.

Jack leaned forward, hoping his close study of the previous night's Alfred Hitchcock film would serve him well. His lips touched Millie's lightly and she melted into him and her mouth opened. Jack jerked back, surprised, but Millie murmured softly against his lips and he opened his mouth and let her tongue explore his. It was incredible, the dance of tongue's, the wetness of her mouth against the cool dryness of her lips and he put his arms around her shoulders and drew her closer to him. For the first time in months the red red red was gone, replaced by a sense of well being and relaxed concentration. The music was quieter too now. His hand came to rest on her back then crawled around to the front of her tee shirt. But Millie had other plans and her hand darted down to his pants and she began to unbutton

34

them.

"Are you sure Millie?" Jack asked hoarsely, as she engulfed him in her sensitive but awkward mouth. Her response was mumbled and the red red red passed into the silky whiteness of her tongue on him and he lay back and forgot what it was exactly that troubled him so much these days because what he had dreamed of paled so swiftly against the reality of Millie Benjamin.

When it was over Millie asked him again, "What's it like, the red red redness of it all."

Jack was startled to realize it had vanished for a brief period. "It was gone for the last few minutes. Can we do it again Millie?"

Life was good and sweet those spring months in Albany when the allergens in the air were restrained against the tender young mucous layers in Jack's nose and Millie was all over him. They explored each others bodies and finally had intercourse when Jack turned fifteen. But it wasn't very good, not as good as it should have been. Jack took forever to come and sometimes he didn't and Millie would wonder what she was doing wrong and Jack would feel inadequate and the red red red would blow bloody bubbles into his mind. But then there were the nights when they sat in a low limbed tree holding each other and kissing each other gently on the lips and cheeks and knowing that they were in love – Romeo and Juliet, except not from feuding families.

At eighteen Jack's behavior quieted down. He had gone into a remission, although he wouldn't know that was the reason for another fifteen years. He started attending Cal and moved into the dorms there. Two months into his first semester he began to publish that series of children's verse which would lead him away from the university to

Los Angeles, where he had dreams of making it in the entertainment business. Millie followed him down and they were married on her eighteenth birthday. Her father screamed, hollered, threatened to disinherit her, and ultimately accepted Jackson as his son in law. Jackson's parents were pleased; they liked Millie, but worried about Jackson's future. On their way down to Los Angeles for Jackson's twenty-eighth birthday they argued in the car about Jackson and his first attempt at a novel. So preoccupied were they that they never saw the fruit truck that hit them, ending their lives.

Jackson and Millie fought frequently after this, Jackson reverting to his old behavior of tics and noises when excited. After a few weeks he made noises all the time including shouting the word 'bitch' at Millie even when they were happy. Millie found herself bewildered by Jackson – he was still Jackson then – and tried to reconnect with him. Her voice lessons were going nowhere, her notes on Jackson's novel only frustrated him, and when their old friend Henry Larkin moved to Santa Monica, an affair began quickly. Millie filed for divorce and as *Lucia* rose on the best seller lists, Jackson's dreams began to erode. The divorce cost him his health and most of the settlement went to lawyers, to Millie, and to the IRS.

Jackson paid his alimony on time. They saw each other on social occasions. They followed the same music, supported the arts, worked the same volunteer functions and in time the pain faded. But the trust that Jackson had found in that first kiss was dead, and no other woman met his first impression and fantasy of Millie Benjamin.

NINE

Dr. Collins listened to Jackson's questions with interest. Jackson had really studied the literature he had been given and had an innate grasp of his disorder. He seemed to connect details of his disorder with the facts and was drawing his own conclusions regarding it. Jackson continued, "But from eighteen to twenty-seven I had virtually no symptoms, just neck tics. I didn't swear or hear colors or anything. Does that make sense, given the diagnosis of Tourette syndrome?"

"Yes. There is some percentage of remissions, not total but during long periods without stress or serious emotional issues the Tourette syndrome symptoms may shut down almost entirely. What happened in your late twenties?"

Jackson looked at Dr. Collins in amazement and began to cry. "Jesus ... I never thought there was a connection. My parents died in a car accident six months after my first novel came out. It was the high point of my life, the book had just entered the national best sellers list, and then within weeks, everything fell apart. They died, my noises came back, my tics got worse and I started to drink very heavily for the first time. You think that's what triggered the return of the Tourette syndrome?"

"Undoubtedly." Dr. Collins paused. "I think that's what is happening now too. The stress of having another best selling book, the tour you're going on next week, these things are pushing you to your limits. The relationship of stress and neurological disorders is a marriage made in hell. How do you feel about possibly going into therapy when you get back from your tour?"

"I don't like the idea at all. I'm not crazy, you told me that." Jackson was defensive but underneath it was something else – fear perhaps, or just embarrassment at his tears. Jackson never cried, that was something Jack had done. More, now than ever, the split between the two periods of his life were growing stronger. Jack the crazy, Jackson the success. But it was Jack who had been in love with Millie, and Jackson who had been alone for seven years, scared to date for embarrassment that his symptoms would act up.

"It's not just for crazy people Jackson. You're under more stress than is normal and your body is showing it. In the three weeks I've known you your tics have doubled, your coprolalia is louder, these sensations you describe sound much worse. I'd like you to at least go on some medication for the symptoms while you're on the road - nothing major, but something to at least just take the edge off."

"An anti-psychotic drug like haloperidol?" Jackson asked nervously, having found the descriptions of the drugs side effects frightening to read.

"No. An anti-anxiety drug or a medication for your obsessive compulsive thoughts. I think it may lower your stress level and also help with the tics and vocal symptoms. What do you think?"

"What are the side effects bitch?"

"Depending on the drug, it can range from dry mouth, blurred vision to muscle spasms, sedation or even impotence. But these side effects are mostly short term and you'll adjust to them over time."

"Gee, impotence. Well, I'm not seeing anybody right now ... The rest I can handle. How would my drinking affect the medication?"

"You should stop. There is an interaction and it may make the side effects worse, particularly the sedation."

"Great. Okay, I'll try the medicine. I'll think about the therapy too."

Dr. Collins nodded, writing a prescription. He was glad that Jackson was agreeable today. "One other thing. You seem very worried about the violent imagery you're obsessing on. I can't reassure you too much about that, but I've never had a Tourette syndrome patient act on these impulses. You may scare yourself with them, that's why I recommended therapy, to deal with the fear. But the chance you'll actually hurt someone is remote."

Jackson smiled. "Bitch it. Thank you for the reassurance Dr. Collins. I know I haven't been the best patient but today helped a lot."

"That's what I'm here for. See you when you get back from your tour?"

"Yes. In five weeks. After the ABA Convention."

"ABA?" Dr. Collins was confused. "The American Bar Association?"

"The American Booksellers Association. It's the big yearly event in publishing."

"Oh. Well, have fun Jackson."

Jackson stood up to go and twitched his neck violently. He held his hand against his head and asked lightly, "It won't fall off will it?"

"Your head? No." Dr. Collins chuckled.

Jackson left and Dr. Collins made some notes for a few minutes. He stopped abruptly and wondered if Jackson would be able to deal with the increasing pressure of being a public figure. Well, he had the right attitude for now. As long as his symptoms were kept under control.

TEN

The colors exploded around Jackson, red red red melting into a fiery orange then expressing itself as a twitch of the neck until the red red red and the fire was relieved. He felt a pulling at his eyes, a crawling almost, like a chill wind, or small insects feasting, and he blinked out of control five times. His mind got stuck on a phrase of Bizet's, but he couldn't place it. He stuck with it though, driving with Sara in the taxi to the airport.

"Damn it!" He shouted, trying to find the words that were haunting him. "Bitch fuck bitch music."

The taxi driver grunted. Jackson grunted back, echoing him, almost like a ritual prayer. The driver grunted again, heard Jackson grunting and turned around in his seat and glared. "Ya imitating me?"

"No. I just ... have this thing, bitch this disorder ... "

"Fuck you."

Jackson blinked five times and turned to Sara. She snarled at the driver, "Watch your lip."

The driver laughed. "I saw this one on *L.A. Law*. Tourist syndrome, yeah, that's what ya got."

Jackson nodded, relieved and mystified. "I'm glad you understand."

Grunt from the driver. Echo from Jackson. "Ya see a lot of it in cabs. People holding in their noises and tics, then finding in a cab a safe place to release it. Like ya."

Jackson had an uncannily weird image of hordes of travelers, outwardly normal, Touretting out in the back of taxi cabs and the drivers, strange foreign men with unheard of accents diagnosing each case through the help of a medical article sent to each and every one of them that drove by their cab companies as a public service.

Jackson also wondered if there was anyone out there who hadn't heard of this rare disorder. "I wonder ..." Jackson got stuck on the phrase and began repeating it over and over again trying to find some way to resolve it. "I wonder I wonder I wonder ..."

The driver came in on top of his words, " ... Who wrote the book of love!"

Jackson laughed. "Echolalia" floated off his tongue to drift in the now still empty silence of the cab. The driver grinned and tore off furiously down the highway to the airport.

Sara clutched at his arm to keep her balance in the cab and whispered to Evans, "You'll keep it under control on the airplane, won't you?"

"I hate to fly, but I can try to suppress it a little."

"You can do that?" Sara asked in surprise.

"At times. I'm still learning how to control it."

"I hope this is one of them – the ABA Show is in two weeks and you're our prime writer to display."

Display. Jackson sucked on the word a moment not liking the taste of it.Hey, it's only a trade show. But the thought of being on display, stared at, mocked! tore into the tender flesh of his unconscious like rats in the eyes of the famine dead.

41

ELEVEN

The flight was Hell – crowded, hot and turbulent. Jackson sat next to the window, his neck twitching very badly under the stress of the lurching movements of the plane. He tore apart his in-flight bag of cholesterol-free peanuts and washed them down with a mini bottle of scotch. He began to mutter loudly to himself, "Bitch, shit, bitch, bitch."

Sara put her hand on his and asked quietly, "Does it get worse when you fly?"

"Shit. Only when I'm stressed out. I didn't sleep last night, I was too wound up taking notes and sketching out some ideas."

Sara smiled at him. "You are back in a writing mode then. Congratulations. So, tell me, what is it about?"

"What? Fuck you. You mean the new book I'm playing with?"

"Playing. What a nice word to hear from you, mister self – obsessed writer ... "

"Bitch. Shit. HEY!"

The stewardess came over to them and said sternly, "You'll have to be quieter, sir. There are children on board."

Sara said to her, "He can't help it."

Jackson said along with her, their voices overlapping, "Fuck you I can't help it."

The stewardess moved off in a huff. Sara looked after

her, a worried look crossing her brow. Jack leaned back and stretched his neck, yelping out loud as he did so. The woman in the seat in front of him turned around to stare. Jackson blew her a kiss and whispered, "Bitch." The woman pressed her call button and leaned her seat back violently, banging Jackson's legs.

"What the Hell's your problem lady, bitch?" Jackson asked pleasantly, his mind on the phrase he had been looking for: Music! what a splendid art, but what a sad profession. Was it Bizet though?

A uniformed man strode up to them, his official attitude lurching along with the plane.

"I'm the co-pilot. The stewardess called me. Is there a problem here?"

"Fuck you. I have Tourette syndrome."

"I'm afraid I don't know what that is sir. Are you in any physical danger?"

"Pardon bitch?"

The co-pilot winced and motioned helplessly at the stewardess. "Give this man a Dramamine. He's going into a seizure or something ..."

"No I'm not," Jackson shouted his neck twitching back violently and causing him to bite down on his tongue. He yelped and the co-pilot saw a drop of blood on his lip.

"Oh Christ. Get the engineer, we'll have to move him upstairs before he lets go." The stewardess ran forward, the co - pilot started fumbling with Jackson's seat belt.

"What the fuck are you doing?" Jackson demanded.

"Are you delirious? How long do we have before you fit?"

"Fit? What am I; a shoe to be tried on? FUCK FUCK BITCH!" Jackson yelled out.

The co pilot motioned to the stewardess. "We'll put

43

him upstairs by himself, his friend can keep an eye on him."

"This is really unnecessary." Sara said angrily, as the engineer pulled at Jackson's legs and the co-pilot pulled on his arms. The woman in front of Jackson began to cry, muttering something about "drunks."

"Regulations miss. If he gets OOC, we want him tied down for the safety of the other passengers."

"OOC?"

"Out of control."

Jackson winced. "What about a Scotch and we forget this whole thing? HEY!"

The co - pilot started frog marching Jackson down the aisle of the plane. With Sara following, they went up the stairs to the upper compartment of the 747, which was empty except for two men drinking bourbon and discussing football scores. "You stay up here, and try not to fit out, okay?" the co - pilot said, starting to sense something was very wrong. Jackson still hadn't gone into a seizure, and was standing up looking menacing. "I don't fit - I have a movement disorder."

The co-pilot headed down the stairs, saying to the stewardess, "I'll have security meet us in Dallas. This guy is very messed up."

The other two passengers in the compartment eyed Jackson warily. Jackson snapped at them, "You heard him, I'm dangerous, beat it."

They did.

Sara sat next to Jackson and held his hand softly in her own. His neck snapped and she whispered to him, "My God dear, what's wrong? I've never seen you this bad."

"I hate to fly. Shit. Hemingway crashed, Glenn Miller crashed, Will bitch Rogers crashed. Why not me?"

"Fear of dying or fear of flying?"

Jackson was startled by the rhyme and froze for a second. "More fear of flying. Death in the abstract I can deal with. Bitch. But death in the air, spinning out of control, flames, shit it's all so real to me - so red."

"Red? You said something about red the other day when we were late to the signing. What do you mean, red like in blood or fire?"

"No, I mean red as an emotion, angry red, abraded red, irritated beyond control, bitch shit red. What I'm feeling inside me right now is red."

"Is this you or your Tourette?"

"I don't know. Just hold me for a moment." Sara backed away slightly, then put her arms around him. "It's not a commitment, just a hug."

Sara held him and after another ten minutes he had calmed down. The co-pilot came back upstairs and glanced at Sara rocking Jackson. "I won't call security. That was just to get you out of the way of the other passengers. I don't fully understand what's wrong with you but it's scary as hell to sit in front of."

"Thank you ... " Sara began.

"Call the fucking Nazi's, you stupid bastard. I'm suing your piss bitch shit airline ... "

"Jack! Shut up for a moment, he's doing you a favor."

"Some favor." Jackson responded bitterly.

The co pilot looked angrily at Jackson. "Your failure to disclose your medical condition is very irresponsible sir ..."

"Disclose? What the hell is wrong with you man, this isn't a yellow star to be wrapped around my arm."

"Jack ... "

"Shut up Sara. Look you asshole, I'm going to sue you for abusive flying."

45

The co-pilot shouted at Jackson, having had enough of his fury, "I'm calling the sky marshals to wait for us in Dallas. Consider yourself under arrest for causing a dangerous situation on an aircraft." He stamped off leaving Jack speechless for the moment.

Sara was crying and Jackson hugged her to him. "I'm sorry bitch."

"We're alone on an airplane. Enjoy it." Sara smoothed down his hair. Oh, she thought, he's starting to bald, just like father ...

Jackson looked at Sara and grinned. "Alone?" He began.

"Perhaps. We'll share a hotel room tonight, if you calm down."

Jackson smiled at her holding her hand tightly. She thought sweetly, he's like a little boy. But I'm a woman and can't let this get out of hand. Once I'm back in New York and he's back in Los Angeles, it's over. Sex is sex and business is business and never the twain shall meet except during ABA month.

Instead of sky marshal's, they were greeted by a representative of the airline, who upon hearing the name of the passenger involved, panicked, and handed Jackson a free roundtrip ticket anywhere in the country. Jackson accepted the apologies with dignity, inwardly relieved that this scene had been avoided. Sara was worried though, wondering when next her writing charge would go off like a rocket.

Jackson was happy though. It was Bizet.

TWELVE

The American Booksellers Association convention is the biggest yearly event in the publishing world. Like the Oscar's or the Grammy's, they represent the superstars of the publishing world with famous writers in attendance. They show off the technical end of things with future projects previewed for the publishing world to talk up. Jackson Evans was scheduled to be the chief guest at the Rockford House cocktail party. Sara was concerned about him even before the ABA Convention opened.

"I don't know Nelson, he's been pretty depressed since the flight and he's drinking a great deal. I don't know how to handle him."

Nelson Rockford, son of the founding publisher and current C.E.O. of Rockford House, laughed at Sara over the hotel room phone. "When I hired you I knew it was a good idea. Just babysit him, tell him he's a good writer, a great speaker and that as soon as he starts his next book we can renegotiate his contract."

"His next book ... He's working on something now, something different."

"Something like *Lucia*? God, I hated that piece of dreck!"

"It made you a lot of money." Sara said, defending

Jackson.

"Yeah, but nobody bought the film rights. That's almost unheard of around here. No paperback deal overseas. But *Backstabbers!*, Lord is that book pulling it in, did you know we're at 450,000 units sold in just four months? Book of the Month Club wants to talk about his next book ..."

"It's about Tourette syndrome."

Nelson laughed nervously. "What is? His next book? God, almighty, he just got diagnosed last month, how can he write a book about it already. Music - that's what he knows about after all those years working for record companies as a publicist. He should do a sequel to *Backstabbers!*, or a new book, maybe a sex and rock and roll twist like Robbins used to write."

"He's outlining it every night."

"Every night? How do you know – My God, you're screwing him! Jesus! Well, keep it quiet, I want the gossip columnists to see him with movie stars, not editorial assistants."

"Thanks a lot Nelson. Fuck you too." Sara hung up.

Nelson looked at his current mistress, who worked for Publishers Weekly, and grinned. "Well, at least she's getting laid for once. That should quiet down the PMS. Where did you put the massage oil?"

THIRTEEN

Sara swore into the phone and thought fondly of Jackson, who was off in his room shaving. So far they hadn't made love, just slept together, his warm hands on her breasts, holding them like delicate eggs, or pearls of great price. Jackson was impotent from his medication, and while Sara had tried to arouse him, it had proven worthless. So they kissed and cuddled and held each other and it was by far nicer than any sex she had ever had. In fact, it was very much like what she pictured an old married couple doing, except that Jackson's twitches as he tried to fall asleep were unexpected at times and last night he had almost thrown her out of bed. But she rubbed his neck for him, and tickled his back and he fell asleep, still talking away about his new writing project.

Sara had never been in intimate contact with a writer at work. Jackson talked about his new book while outlining it – while eating – while giving her head, he would mutter ideas to her, causing her to giggle hysterically. But he was like a man possessed, and his drinking had started to get under control, with Jackson writing most of the morning on yellow legal pads, scrawling his outline and chapter drafts. Sara was transcribing it into her laptop computer and having the floppy disc's printed out by Rockford House every few days. Then Jackson would make corrections on the printouts, he would read the scenes out loud to her - God! it was so intimate to hear it first - then she would make the required changes, send off the revised disc and to her amazement, Jackson was already, after only two weeks, fifty pages into the first draft. She loved his energy but feared evenings when he went to autograph parties for *Backstabbers!*, and drank too much to hide his embarrassment at being a public figure.

People magazine had written a profile on him, the disabled best selling writer, and while he was internally complimented, outside he was full of scorn and cynicism.

Sara loved it all. Jackson had decided to come out of the closet about his Tourette syndrome, following the example of baseball player Jim Eisenreich and basketball pro Chris Jackson. There was a long tradition of literary figures with Tourette-like disorders: Samuel Johnson with his obsessive rituals and twitches, Andre Malraux with his involuntary vocalizations, and the stammering Emperor Claudius of Rome who had written an Etruscan Dictionary. So Jackson felt he had good role models and a valuable service to provide to younger people with Tourette syndrome. But the psychic cost to Jackson, meeting all the questions of the media, the bad reporting, the snickers when he drank too much and people wondered if it was his Tourette Syndrome that drove him to drink (It was, it wasn't. It was mostly trying to obliterate the steadily increasing images of violence and red red red he saw in his mind, intruding all the time now.) Jackson almost regretted being public about it. But when he looked at his new manuscript and saw the insights that his writing was giving him about himself, he felt better about it.

What he didn't feel good about was being back in a relationship. Sex after Millie was no sex at all. Millie had been able to arouse him like no other woman could, and while he liked Sara and was quite attracted to her, he just couldn't get an erection around her. It was strange, but this morning while shaving he had gotten hard but by the time he had found Sara in the breakfast lounge he was impotent again. He wondered if it was the medication or something else, something inside him which said he couldn't have a woman the way normal men could. He didn't know and to a degree didn't want to know.

FOURTEEN

The cocktail party given by Rockford House for *Backstabbers!* was very much in demand after Jackson's performance on the airplane trip was reported by Entertainment Tonight. People were begging for invitations and when Sara ran out mid afternoon, invitations actually went on the black market with people selling them for fifty bucks or trading them in for a chance to hear James Michener talk about his 'little' book on the universe he was planning in twelve volumes.

Gossip swirled around the ABA Convention like so many dust motes caught in an updraft or tiles falling off the space shuttle on a descent into the Earth's atmosphere. Rockford House was getting good press: *Backstabbers!* was the most discussed book of the year. Jackson Evans was now richer than before – Rockford House was the nation's fastest growing hardback house – and Sara wondered if Jackson could handle the additional fame. Of course if he couldn't, Nelson Rockford could always buy another writer from another publishers and sell potboilers instead of fine literature. But Nelson was typical of the new rich – the new publishing – the new post yuppie greedheads who were turning publishing into an adjunct of Hollywood, where every book had to be made into a movie to be considered successful.

Jackson Evans had other plans.

In his notes on his new book, a semi-autobiographical novel about Tourette syndrome, he had made the comment that, "What was unsaid by the general public was often the first words out of the mouth of somebody with Tourette syndrome.

You need a honest man, look for someone with Tourette syndrome to tell it like it is, for in a world drowning in pollution, medical malpractice, and the politics of greed, people who couldn't control their words were the rarity. A million glowing Ronald Reagan's on the campaign trail except they knew words the Gipper didn't."

Jackson had an unusual framework for his novel – it dealt with the classical search by Diogenes for a honest man and what the reaction was when the world found out he was disabled by some strange cursing disorder. It was allegorical, of course, which was out of fashion, and it was planned to be very short, under 200 pages, which most publishing houses hated. They wanted books that were medium sized so they could charge $19.95 for about $1.50 of paper and cardboard, ripping off the general public by pretending they were getting ART instead of the usual 'screw 'em again' trash that filled the best seller lists in New York and Los Angeles, two cities where more people got raped than had read a book in a year.

FIFTEEN

The cocktail party given by Rockford House was totally packed, and when Jackson and Sara arrived, fashionably late of course, it took them over twenty minutes to get in. Security checks at the door, handing over their invitations, coat racks to be fought over for a space, all the usual things one does at a corporate party. Jackson was dying for a drink but Sara had other plans. She led him to various executives of Rockford House where he could be fawned over, satisfying his ego but not quenching his thirst. Al Fredericks, Nelson's second in command, had an idea for a follow up to *Backstabbers!* about a diva in the recording world. Jackson pointed out that he had already written about opera and the recording world and had no interest in writing again about either. Al got squirrelly looking – he actually resembled a ferret – and apologized. Jackson snuck off after an hour and got a beer.

Nelson Rockford was in a good temper. He played with his glasses, touched his upper lip repeatedly where he had shaved his mustache that morning for the party, and eyed the women in the room compulsively. He sat next to

Sara on a couch and asked her if she was having a good time.

"Yes. You?"

"Real happy. We're going public next quarter, might even sell the company off to Yoshi Yoshihara if he wants it. I could then do what I dreamed of since I was fifteen."

"Which is what?" Sara asked.

"Nothing. Just ride my horses, love my wife and eat Chinese food upon occasion. The relaxed life."

"Oh." Sara was always appalled by the emptiness of her boss' mind, it seemed that there should be more there, some deep thought beyond sex and food, but it never came out. The fact of the matter was, Nelson Rockford was in his tenth year of therapy, and liked to wear rubber garments to bed.

He could afford it now.

Jackson tossed back another beer – his third – and listened to the milling conversation in the crowded hotel suite. All around the crowded room he saw famous writers and those who wrote about famous writers and those who were not famous but merely rich. Conversations drifted red red red through his ears, fragments of arguments about current books, stock market yields, movies, and of course, what the Reagan's were up to now that Ronnie had returned to acting. Had he ever really stopped, Jackson wondered outloud, then began to listen to the conversations around him.

"I wonder if anybody reads anymore."

"I read this graffiti last week in New York ... "

"Graffiti! What about the new Ford ad ... "

"Ford? You must be joking. Harlan Ellison is doing another series of ads for GEO ... "

"GEO was a nice magazine but who wants to look at

pictures of dying animals ... "

"Animal? I hear he was almost thrown off the plane from Dallas ... "

This sounded interesting, and Jackson wondered how word of it had leaked so fast. (Nelson, upon hearing of it, had issued a press release. You never knew what would help sales ...)

"He was drunk and swearing and groping this poor stewardess. Luckily they knocked him unconscious with a bottle of wine and he is now fucking the editorial assistant who worked on his last book."

That wasn't in the press release but Sara and Jackson were sharing a hotel room. Jackson was impotent, but after all, sex was dangerous these days so it might be for the best. Sara hadn't made love in six months, and still went in for regular HIV blood tests. She almost wanted to get AIDS so she would have an '90's type of excuse for celibacy.

... And not fall in love with Jackson ...

"I heard this great joke. What do you call shake and bake?"

"I don't know, what?"

"Jackson Evans cooking!"

The group laughed. Jackson headed for the other end of the room, away from the glitter and closer to the writing crowd. A famous rock star had just shown up with a guitar and was singing some of his more obscure songs, with a crooning tenderness that age brings to men with bad voices. Seated at his feet was a bearded man with a paunch who looked familiar to Jackson. It took him a moment to place him, but then he did. It was Oliver Sacks, M.D. the neurologist turned writer who had written *Awakenings* and was considering writing a whole volume on Tourette syndrome from an anthropological point of view. Jackson waved him over and Sacks bounded up to him cheerfully, white beard displaying remnants of his lunch.

"Mr. Evans! Ah ... a pleasure. I ... ah ... wanted to talk to you about an interview."

"The pleasure bitch is mine. I hear we're writing about the same thing fuck these days."

"Ah ... the Tourette, you mean? Good good, you should write about it in your own way."

"You don't fear the competition?"

"Robert De Niro did my last film too. Ah ... You seem so ill at ease by these things ... do you hate parties as much as me?"

"More so. Let's go down to the hotel coffee shop and talk bitch."

Sacks smiled, delighted and pulled out a notebook and a blue pen. "Bitch is one of your vocal symptoms, then?"

"That and other words. Bitch fuck whore shit."

"Was that a list or a tic?"

"Both." The two writers grinned at each other and Sacks put away his notebook, reached into his pocket for a handkerchief, reached into his other pocket to put away his pen, found an orange there and tossed it from hand to hand while talking away in a British tinged stammer. Jackson was delighted.

SIXTEEN

"Publishing sucks." Jackson announced at the final morning press conference when talking about the problems of breaking into print.

All in all, everybody else on the panel agreed and left to catch their flights back home where they could slave over their next novel with the hopes of a multimillion dollar advance or an option from the movies.

Jackson went to the nearest bar and ordered a Long Island iced tea. "To Steinbeck," he toasted, and drank it down. He looked at the bearded bartender, and said quietly, "That was the last drink of my life."

"Ya quitting?"

"Yeah. I gotta book to write and I need to be sober to do it."

"Good luck." The bartender stared at the open ABA Convention program and glanced at Jackson. "Say, didn't you write that opera book?"

"Yeah." Jackson felt smugly delighted - everybody had read *Lucia* it seemed.

"It stank. God, haven't you ever been to Italy? Shit,

you described La Scala like a Vegas Bordello."

Jackson laughed. "It was my first novel."

"How'd it sell?"

"Too well. People like trash for some reason. My next book's going change all that, set people back on edge over a work of fiction."

The bartender nodded. "Yeah, Gore Vidal said that last night too."

Jackson laughed once, then stopped, silenced in thought.

SEVENTEEN

Over the next few months things settled into a regular routine. With the profits from *Backstabbers!* Jackson bought a nice new two bedroom house in the San Fernando Valley, in spitting distance, literally, (it was a new tic) from Ventura boulevard. He set the second bedroom up as a writing office with two large wooden desks and a huge bulletin board with his outline and various notes. On one desk were stacks of three by five cards, yellow legal pads and three jars of pencils. On the other desk was an IBM Computer and printer and three reams of 20 pound bonded paper. On the walls were photographs of Monterey harbor and a collage of down beat Magazine's 55th anniversary cover.

Mornings he wrote, afternoons he read Dos Passos or

Hemingway and made notes on their technique, some evenings he went to continental jazz clubs like Le Cafe or Bon Appetit to hear fusion groups trying to play the most notes in the fastest amount of time. They were so loud that Jackson's noises didn't bother anyone. Certain groups seemed to be defining a new sound; a blend of fusion and New Age that Jackson found interesting to study. Jackson kept sober, at least most of the time, although when the writing went bad, he would kick back a shot or two of Cuervo Gold Tequila. But that was increasingly rare these days.

After five months, *The Honest Man* was approaching the end of its first draft and Sara called Jackson every day for an update. Even though they were yet to make love successfully, things had settled into a semblance of a relationship with Sara's morbid fear of AIDS kept calm by this form of bicoastal monogamy. Jackson wrote her little poems now and then and would mail them to her in his huge scrawling handwriting.

He had a secretary now, twenty two year old punk rocker Maggie Ryan, who transcribed the yellow pages onto computer and FAXED them to Sara – For Her Eyes Only – every Friday morning. Weekends Sara would edit and comment and discuss the book with Jackson. Jackson loved the way the book was going, felt he had finally broken through the shell of superficiality that had so marred his earlier fiction. Sara encouraged him, but felt differently about the book.

She hated it.

It was first of all, very serious and pompous, bloated with Jackson's personal sense of outrage and fury at God for having given him Tourette syndrome. The book was short, incredibly slow moving and had no specific character

59

names. Instead there was the honest man (the presidential candidate) the beggar (The incumbent party head) the son of God (George Bush) and the fallen woman (Jesse Jackson). The usage of Tourette syndrome in the book with the honest man swearing and telling everybody what he thought climaxed about fifty pages before the end, which was a recapitulation of the first two hundred pages. Sara honestly didn't get what the book was trying to say. It was set during a presidential convention but was filled with biblical and classical allusions that were confusing and extremely arbitrary.

Sara couldn't tell any of this to Jackson over the phone – not while he was still writing. Nelson had inquired about the manuscript but Jackson wanted to give him a completed book, rather than a sample chapter and outline. Nelson bitched and whined, but with *Backstabbers!* at one million copies in world wide sales, he really didn't give a damn. Negotiations with Yoshihara were going well; the SEC had no objections to Rockford House going public and Nelson had bought an inflatable doll that looked just like Barbara Cartland. Life was good and sweet.

EIGHTEEN

After the People magazine story broke, Jackson began receiving fan mail at Rockford House from other people with Tourette syndrome. The letters followed several typical patterns: Some were congratulatory, others asked for money as 'Brothers in Tourette'. One Jackson kept on his office bulletin board for a month, then finally answered it. It read:

Dear Mr. Evans,

My name is Jason Watkins and I am nine years old. I want to be a writer. You are my hero. I have had my Tourette since the age of six and although it has hurt me, other people have hurt me more. My mom runs the Monterey Tourette Rap Group. She has Tourette, too. We were diagnosed together, and I love my mother because she understands me better than any other person in the world. I think you would understand me too. I read your first novel, but mom wouldn't let me read your second book because she said it was too dirty. I looked at a few pages of it at the book store and I think she was right. But I want to read it. You are my favorite writer. If you aren't too busy, please write back.

Love,
Jason Watkins

Jackson sent Jason Watkins an autographed copy of *Backstabbers!* and a note saying:

Dear Jason,

Wait until your mom thinks you're old enough to read this. Your letter meant a lot to me, coming from a fellow writer. Keep up the fight!

Jack

Jackson started going to AA meetings about once a week. Dr. Collins had recommended them and Jackson was curious to see other alcoholics at close range. He wasn't sure he wanted the title alcoholic but saying he had a drinking problem was like saying that Dan Quayle was a little dependent on his father. Like Quayle he needed his crutch, and when he drank his tics calmed down somewhat, and he could forget for a little while the pain that was causing him to drink.

He didn't want to be recognized so he wore a lowslung sombrero and an overcoat. People who saw him at the AA meetings thought he was a Mexican flasher. When sober, Jackson had retained his strange sense of the dramatic and would bring one of a series of carved animal shaped pipes that he had bought second hand at a garage sale in Whittier. Jackson hadn't totally stopped drinking, but on good days when the words came cleanly and with an element of honesty he was able to go without alcohol. On those nights he went to AA and observed quietly, not participating but feeling comforted by the group experience. Occasionally someone would comment on his tics, but for the most part he felt secure there. Once he came close to saying "My name is Jack and I'm an aAlcoholic" but he found the thought too disturbing to actually follow through on. The idea of going public with a vice – to be revealed as imperfect before a group of strangers repelled him. But he found comfort in watching the other people follow the AA ritual and he read the handouts and, during the social period following the meetings, he would unwind and talk to some of the other drunks and try to share his pain with them one on one.

Over the course of the summer he stopped drinking entirely for three weeks, then hit a snag in the middle of the book and went down for a bender. It was one of those dark nights that you can't quite forget and can't quite remember. After the vomit was cleaned up, he called Sara and broke down over the phone.

"I need you."

"I can't leave New York right now; we're in preproduction on five books."

"Then I'm coming to New York. I'm dying out here fuck. I ... want to be with you again."

"How's our little problem?"

"The drinking or the impotency?"

"The drinking is your problem. I meant the other." Sara felt ashamed at her coldness but this call wasn't like the other ones recently from Jackson. He sounded so scared and lonely, so in need of her that she was frightened by his intensity. As long as he was the fun little boy she knew from the book tour she felt safe. But to bring real feelings into it frightened Sara.

"I had an erection last night."

"I hope you didn't waste it."

Jackson laughed. "No, I didn't." He paused then said softly, "it had your name on it."

Sara was silent for a long moment that stretched out until Jackson thought they had been disconnected. He said "Hello?"

"Would you want to stay with me?"

"Yes, if you didn't mind."

"I haven't been with anyone since the book tour - God I'd love to see you! This weekend?"

"Yes. I ... I mean ... I love you Sara."

"I see."

"That's it, I see?"

"I can't commit as easily as you Jack. But I do care deeply about you."

"Care deeply? Jesus Sara, that's how people feel about saving the dolphin or little children. We spent three weeks sharing a bed, a life, a vision, and you can't tell me how you feel about me. What the Hell is pushing you away?"

"I'm not pushing you away."

"Meaning what? That I am?"

"Maybe. Look Jack, this is happening so fast ... "

"Fast? God damn it it's been five months now. Look, I'll have Maggie FAX you the flight information and we'll thrash this thing out in person. Love you. Bye."

Sara stared at the phone in frustration, having wanted to get the last word in. Control was a bitter God to worship. But worship it she did. She wondered how she felt about Jack, did she really love him, or did she love the fact that they hadn't yet had intercourse and he still wanted her. Life was weird in the 1990's – sex was even weirder and Sara desperately wanted to make soft gentle love to him, and make him whole again sexually. She wondered what damage his wife had caused him and wondered what he would say if he found out that she was psychologically a virgin. She wasn't really – at a Vassar mixer she had been with a Harvard man whose name she never knew, but she hadn't had a total sexual experience since then. What did she feel about her relationship with Jack and why did men have to have penises? Life was so complex.

NINETEEN

With pen in hand I write
Not knowing if I am right,
Or wrong about my words
That flow out of me like turds.

In the morning it's RUSH RUSH RUSH
Trying to accomplish so damn much
In so little time - so little time.

Words phrases honor
Sex violence truth
These are my Gods - my soul
My words of work - my goal.

First draft revisions
Marred by visions,
Of rejection from the readers
My words to the hungry needers.

Second draft blues
Writers Guild dues
Incoming royalties

Echolalia

Outgoing frailties.

Final draft the big edit
Screaming fight - I've just had it
Proof sheets of bloody mistakes
Correct them - then escape.

Into the bottle I crawl
Retreat surrender I bawl
Until the book is real
I have no life; just a deal.

Reviews excerpts interviews
The bullshit of the market
Everybody has a separate view
The writer is an open target.

I read I write
I drink I think
For those are my working days
And these are my working nights

Words without end Amen
Bury me at the end
And write on my headstone,
In words of timeless gray –

"He was read without a groan,
But now he's gone – silently,
Like his life, and only
His books remain."

TWENTY

Jackson flew Delta Airlines with Maggie, who had never been to New York. Rockford House was supplying him with an empty office and he was going to finish the first draft there, then submit it to Nelson. Sara met them at the airport, waiting in the crowded dirty terminal at Kennedy. She was aware of the dirt and the people crushing around her. She was scared about seeing Jackson again. It would require her to feel, and right now she didn't want feelings, she wanted to be the impartial editor. Jackson saw Sara first and walked up to her. She flung her arms around him and they kissed.

"This is Maggie. This is Sara, my inspiration, the only honest woman in publishing!"

Sara laughed self consciously, and they began walking to the baggage counter, following the rest of the empty headed travelers who were grateful for their escape from the turbulence and the endless descriptions by the honey voiced pilot from Kansas of natural wonders on the opposite side of the airplane.

In New York Jackson set Maggie up at the Hotel

Olcott, a residential hotel on West 72nd that catered mostly
to musicians. Simultaneously with his arrival, the paperback rights of *Backstabbers!* sold for a record amount due
to the film tie in. Jackson was now a millionaire – at least
on paper (or in paper, depending on how you looked at
things) – and Maggie immediately asked for a raise. Jackson turned her down but did establish a CD redeemable in
five years in her name, assuming she finished out the new
book with him. Maggie desperately wanted to go back to
Los Angeles, shave her head and start a punk rock band, but
shortly she was taken with New York and never mentioned
the raise again.

Besides, Nelson Rockford was slipping her a thousand
dollars a week to look secretly at the manuscript.

Jackson started buying odd gifts for those close in his
life; a life sized stuffed carousel horse from FAO Schwartz
was delivered to Sara's apartment one fine Saturday morning to her delight and the neighbors horror. Jackson had a
photographer in that afternoon to take pictures of the two of
them mounted on the horse and Nelson leaked his copy to
the press the following week. News of their affair was now
public. For Nelson, Jackson bought a life sized figure by
Sally Lewis, the San Rafael artist, of a dirty old man in a
trenchcoat. Nelson proudly put it in his office, next to the
petrified walrus penis that Melvin Belli had given him.

Sex between Jackson and Sara was fairly good, but
unconventional, considering that Jackson had yet to have
an orgasm with Sara except when masturbated by her
expert hands. Sara was comfortable with this except when
she froze up, which she often did. Then Jackson would
gently massage her feet, her ankles and her thighs bringing
her to an insatiable level of arousal then stop abruptly to
read Steinbeck or Faulkner to her. For some reason this

interruption relaxed her enough that when they made love later on that evening she was able to achieve the pleasure she seeked, and that Jackson so lovingly gave. They tried intercourse but were unsuccessful at it together, Jackson going soft or Sara too tense to unwind. They became experts at oral sex, inventing new variations involving ice cubes, ice cream and chocolate syrup.

Nelson Rockford was satisfied as well. The first sales of Rockford House stock would begin the following month and the announcement of a new Jackson Evans novel would definitely raise the price of the new shares. Billionaire publishing kingpin Yoshi Yoshihara had offered to buy 49 percent of the first offering. Two new writers, graduates of the UC Irvine Masters Program, were busy cleaning up their first novels which in a unique move were going to be published together as part of Rockford House's *New Voices* series of novels which would feature introductions by Jackson Evans. The writer knew nothing about this yet, but the news was quietly being leaked and Nelson's new mistress was writing a piece for the New York Times Review of Books about the heavyweight endorsing the two novices. Life was sweet and good.

There was one hang up in Nelson's mind though: He didn't like *The Honest Man* and hoped that on the rewrite Jackson would introduce some additional sex and violence. But until it was officially submitted, he kept quiet, making innocuous comments to Sara when she presented him with weekly progress reports on the upcoming novels in preparation. The previous five books released by Rockford House had done moderately well – 50,000 in sales or so – but it was the next year's lineup that Nelson was banking on. That and the potential of selling off his two novices contract's after their first books (or book) came out.

In October Jackson finished the first draft of *The Honest Man*. After a week of cleaning up the manuscript, he stopped writing for the first time in seven months, with a 200 page book ready for comments from Sara, Nelson and the editorial staff of Rockford House. Jackson celebrated by catching the Chick Corea Akoustic Band at the Blue Note, and having his first drink in three months. Sara and Maggie joined him and they were mentioned in Liz Smith's column the following day. Jackson was often mentioned in the gossip columns because of his best selling book and his increased Tourette syndrome symptoms. Jackson had started taking medication for his Tourette vocalizations prior to evenings out, but refused to take it daily because it clouded his mind too much and worsened his impotency problems. So sometimes while in public he blurted out loud obscenities, or made so much noise at lunches that Sara had to find a private booth when they met for meals. Nelson didn't give a damn – in two months he could buy a restaurant. But being a public figure was becoming increasingly stressful for Jackson, and every few days he would anxiously call Dr. Collins for advice. One week Jackson would try to cut out caffeine but the medication made him groggy and when he drank too much coffee he needed a drink at night to unwind. One drink led to another so he needed more coffee in the morning to fight a hangover. A vicious cycle was born.

Jackson decided to drive up to Woods Hole Port and catch a ferry to Martha's Vineyard while awaiting Rockford House's reaction to *The Honest Man*. Jackson had never been there but a number of articles and books over the years about the island had intrigued him. Sara couldn't get away from her editorial duties at the moment, and Jackson missed her terribly, but he felt they needed time away from each other. During the drive he listened to seven hours of each other. During the drive he listened to seven hours of fusion jazz on his new portable CD player; stopping each hour to drink eight ounces of orange juice and smoke his pipe in the quietness of the early New England autumn. His Tourette syndrome symptoms were under more control for the most part, except for occasional intrusive thoughts about sex, violence or dirt. His neck still twitched constantly – it was his most faithful companion.

In Martha's Vineyard, Jackson stayed at a tiny two room bed and breakfast that faced the harbor in Vineyard Haven and he watched the surf calling to him to drink the sea froth like bubbles in a diet Pepsi. The view from the window was haunting and the first night there Jackson sat entranced as the sunset shimmered off the eastern seaboard. The owner of the B & B had no idea of who Jackson was, and the anonymity was a relief after months of being fawned over in New York.

Jackson spent a lot of time in cemeteries while on the Vineyard exploring tombstones. He was considering a historical novel about the whaling days, but found himself unexpectedly shocked by the tombstones of children, reflecting the high infant mortality rate from the 1700's to the present. His obsession with famine and drought deaths seemed to tune into this, and his notes took on a different colored tinge, not a modern day *Moby Dick* as a theme, but a novel about family tragedy, particularly when he found out through researching at the mariner's exchange that one captain had lost ten children over a twenty year period, and upon his final return with his crew had brought cholera to the island from the China Seas killing off most of his crew, his remaining children and his wife, but he himself survived for ten more years in great pain. Jackson had found his next book, or least the first thread of it.

71

Evenings Jackson ate at little seafood restaurants, or visited friends in Edgartown by the Chappaquidic Bridge. The Kennedy's had extended him an open invitation to visit as had Carly Simon, but Jackson preferred being with people who accepted him as a regular guy instead of a celebrity. He drank little, keeping for the most part sober, but internally was higher than he had been for years. In talking to Sara he found her guarded about the Rockford House reaction, but put that down to her natural caution. He worried briefly about it, but was then invited to visit some of the native American's in Gayhead and off he went to further research his next planned book.

One Indian woman, whose family had lived in the Vineyard for three hundred years was, oddly enough, married to a reformed Rabbi, and the couple made a deep impression on Jackson. That people from totally different backgrounds could come together and find love and happiness made him feel more secure about Sara and himself, even though their differences were medical and emotional, not religious and racial.

But differences there were, and all the love in Jackson Evans' body couldn't seem to reach the ache in Sara's soul, the emptiness left from someone or something in her past. Her inability to trust, to commit was very male – for sake of no other word – and Jackson found it ironic in a way that he had found a macho woman.

Jackson was rethinking their relationship during this visit, wondering what it was he wanted from Sara. He wanted her to love him the way he loved her, but was part of his love the fact that she couldn't love him? Or was it more twisted - was she so much like Millie: Bright, athletic, artistic but emotionally dead? Jackson didn't know, he just knew he was getting to the end of his patience with her.

They had lived together for eights weeks now, their sex life was okay except for the lack of intercourse, they had plenty of friends in New York, they were both working hard and enjoying themselves. So what was missing? Maybe it was too easy, too superficial for Jackson. He liked challenge, thrived on it, and the lack of stress in their relationship made him wonder if there was one. Besides, it didn't seem to be going anywhere, getting more serious or heading towards any kind of commitment on Sara's part.

So what was there?

TWENTY ONE

Jackson's contract with Rockford House was based on the sale of *Lucia* and an option on his second novel *Backstabbers!* In publishing parlance it was a right of first refusal, which, had it been employed, would have made Rockford House a laughing stock for refusing one of the bestselling books of the 1990's. Now Nelson Rockford was up against the wall again, because while Jackson Evans was loyal (so far) to Rockford House, there was no option on the current book. Nelson could pass on *The Honest Man*, and save his house a lot of money from the expected promotional costs for a book that Nelson expected to bomb. But if another house were to pick it up, and the book were to sell, it would damage Rockford House's credibility at a very sensitive time in its history. Nelson was not a Pascal Covici, loyal to his writers, profit or not. But he also wasn't prepared to be laughed at by Publishers Weekly the year he went public. It was a tight call.

Al Fredericks, his editor in chief, and second in command at Rockford House had suggested that Nelson pass on the novel. "It's the dullest fucking book I've ever read. What's happened, has he become a Rebo or something?"

"Rebo?"

"Born again Christian. I swear, there are more references to God in this book than in the Bible ... "

"But it has got a love story, a race riot, politics ... "

"It has got no sale written all over it. I'm not going to go over your decision Nelson, but after next month you've got stockholders to answer to for bad decisions, and Yoshi Yoshihara doesn't like fuckups."

Nelson lit an incense stick in his office and inhaled shallowly. Should he show the book to Yoshihara, get his opinion? No way, he'd just take credit if it sold. He called Sara to his office on the ninth floor of the Manhattan office building that was the chief asset of Rockford House after its catalog of books.

"Sara, I need your opinion. Should we release *The Honest Man*?"

Sara was stunned by the question. While she personally disliked the book, the thought that Rockford House wouldn't publish it had never occurred to her. She stared at Nelson and wondered if kinky sex made men more stupid (or if stupid men just liked kinky sex.)

"How could we pass on such a hot property? The follow up novel by the author of *Backstabbers!* should make publishing history."

"If it's set up right. The book stinks, Sara, you have to agree with that."

Sara nodded grimly. "I do. In its present state."

"Would Jackson work with you to make the mandatory revisions needed - more action, less sermons, and lose the religious themes?"

Sara looked down at the floor. "I don't think he would be willing to make those kind of changes Nelson."

Nelson saw a glorious opportunity to pass the buck. "Okay Sara, here's how we're going to play it. It's in your court whether or not this book comes out with our imprint. You're the editor. If Jackson is willing to make ALL the required changes suggested by our staff, I'll take the chance and publish it. If not - fuck him."

Sara knew she was being set up but also knew it was part of her job. Regardless of what happened, if the book was rejected or revisions forced on Jackson, she suspected that their relationship was over. "I'll talk to Jack when he gets back tonight."

"Give him a kiss for me," Nelson snickered obnoxiously and Sara walked out of his office, cheeks burning hot as if they had just been slapped.

TWENTY TWO

Sara took a long walk that afternoon and thought about loyalties. She loved Jackson, to a degree; after all how much could one truly love in this world and still keep your sense of proportion? She had read all the right magazine articles on selfish men and co - dependency and all the other buzz words that had replaced what used to be called common sense. But she also knew if she blew this one, Rockford House would probably not promote her to full editor, even though she was already performing the functions of one. Should a creative writer be dictated to in order to satisfy salespeople who were not creative? Should she use her love affair with Jackson to cause that forcing? What kind of person would she be if she did?

If she didn't push Jackson she might be unemployed – not the kind of person she wanted to be right now in her life. Jackson would help her out – but she wouldn't take his money, in fact she was supporting him in terms of a roof over his head while he was in New York. But that was quid pro quo, he had paid for all those expensive steak dinners at Smith & Wollensky's.

Loyalties. The word buzzed around her like perverse little demons around the head of George Bush, or flies in the sand at Coney Island where she had grown up. Loyalties. Her job was important – damn it, it was hers! She had

76

fought for it. She was good at it and if she couldn't work with a stubborn writer to make some revisions ... a writer she was sleeping with ... in love with ... oh God it was so confusing!

But all relationships were confusing. That's the essence, the mystery that propels us into them. In therapy that evening she spoke about Jackson in the third person so much that Dr. Lindsay said gently, "Have you already disassociated from him?"

"What do you mean?"

"He's no longer Jack – he's the writer or that damn man I'm fucking, which incidentally you're not."

"We make love." Sara said defensively. "It might seem like foreplay to you but it means a lot to me."

"I'm not saying it doesn't, but it does seem funny how you won't commit to Jack either physically or emotionally. You just seem to keep him at a certain distance then you run away."

Sara mused over that while taking a taxi home. The cab driver tried to flirt with her, but she wasn't paying attention. She sat in her apartment alone, staring at her stuffed horse and wondering what it was she really felt.

The answer came to her in a burst of sudden insight: Nothing.

She felt empty inside and realized that was what she had become after two years at Rockford House - Nelson's twin sister. She started to cry, then thought about his stock portfolio and laughed instead. Then she watched a Robert Redford movie on TV.

TWENTY THREE

Jack drove in about midnight, high as a kite over some new project. Except for the eagerly awaited editorial comments and proof sheets, he had put *The Honest Man* to bed in his own mind and was anxious to get on with his next book. It took Sara an hour to get him to listen to her and he stared at her in shock.

"I couldn't possibly make those changes Sara. They would change the whole tone of the book. It's an allegorical tale, not a 'screw em again' novel. Damn it bitch I want it to be very moral, nothing else is being written today with a semblance of morality; just immorality and death." Jackson felt a red red red glow on his face and touched his chin carefully where he had cut himself shaving that morning. The cut was abraded from constant handling and Jackson knew he was obsessing on it too much. What else was that shade of red; what else held such life in it but blood?

"Jack, listen to me. Nelson will reject your book. Word will get out about this. It will be a very hard book to sell. You will be without a new publishing contract. You may lose your agent. You may lose ... me."

There, it was out. Sara stared at him realizing that in not making a decision she had made one.

Jackson reached for her hand and held it a moment, then picked up his suitcase. "I'll be at the Hotel Olcott if you need me for anything, Ms. Madison. Goodnight."

Jackson left the apartment and Sara waited for the tears to come. They sat behind her eyes, building up but refusing to budge. She tried crying, forcing them out like they taught at acting school. Finally she took a Valium and went to bed.

TWENTY FOUR

When Jackson showed up at Maggie Ryan's suite at three in the morning, he was a broken man inside. Maggie sensed this and also sensed her meal ticket had come in. She undressed him, put him to bed and crawled in after him. But Jackson wasn't interested in sex, only comfort, and Maggie was a cold little bitch who knew lots about the first but was blind to the second.

Jackson awoke the next morning to find Maggie sitting in the living room with a pot of coffee. She was dressed in a light terry cloth bathrobe and her hard pink nipples showed through the fabric. Jackson remembered the night before and felt embarrassed. He also felt horny, and sat down beside her. She poured him a cup of coffee, with sweet and low and steamed milk, the way he liked it, and stared intently into his eyes. He stared at her, thinking deep dark thoughts about sodomy, rape and various forms of forced entry. She looked at him and licked her lips seductively. He moved away from her and she reached out for him. His control snapped and suddenly he was on top of her, untying her robe, her hands eagerly at his pants, pulling down the zipper, reaching for it, lips tightly pressed together, their tongues in rapid motion, my God he's entering her, she's dry but not caring, he's coming, she's moaning and suddenly it's over - finished like a wet dream or a blow job through a hole in a brothel's wall.

"I'm fucking sorry Maggie ... "

"It was ... interesting. I wondered when you would want to lay me. Next time we'll slow down a bit, move a little slower."

"Yeah ... sure. I gotta go ... I'm meeting my agent at ten."

"Screw'em and leave'em." Maggie laughed at the cliche, then stopped suddenly, unsure of what she had gotten herself into.

"I'll be back. Tonight. Dinner?"

"Okay."

TWENTY FIVE

Bernard Crawford was one of New York's most powerful agents. He didn't get there by being a nice guy and when Jackson started to tell him about how his book was being raped by Rockford House and that he wanted a new publishing deal, Bernie looked at him coldly.

"They've offered you an advance of two hundred thousand for the completed manuscript."

"Who has? Rockford? I won't take it."

Bernie cracked his knuckles and thought of the Marquis De Sade - what an agent he would have made! "Jack, you're going to take it or you're going to get the fuck out of my agency. You have a chance to sell a lot of books – why fuck that up with a little integrity?"

"I thought they were going to turn the book down without revisions?"

"They want some – they're faxing them over at noon. You can make the changes, Jack, you will make the changes, it shouldn't be too hard. Then you can write a real book, a sequel to *Backstabbers!* maybe."

Jackson tried to sort this all through his head but his mind was wandering. Why had Sara told him that they were going to reject the book? Was it just a reason to end their relationship? Jackson didn't know, nor did he know why he had practically raped Maggie that morning. Things were too much in flux right now, too red red red and he wanted to go home to Los Angeles and sleep a million nights ...

"Jack, pay some fucking attention."

Jackson looked up and twitched his neck and back violently. Bernard blinked and muttered, "Great, now he's getting more Touretty on me. Look Jack, who told you that the book was going to be rejected?"

"Sara."

"Do you really think they're going to reject your book this week? Did you see Publishers Weekly yesterday? Rockford House goes public on Friday. You're the center of their sales of stock my boy. You can ask for the moon here and get it, fight them over the revisions, and even possibly win. After the stock sale settles down, let them do whatever the fuck they want." Bernard lowered his voice. "I hear Yoshihara's buying in as a silent partner, forty nine percent of the stock. He likes you Jack, you could get that turd Nelson fired if you play your cards straight."

"He owns the house!"

"Until Friday. Then it's Yoshihara's game, and he doesn't like losers. Don't be a loser Jack, be a winner. Sell your book to Rockford before the offering, and demand shares in the house. You'll be set for life – I know several people who would like to buy in, buy your shares at market value as of Friday."

"Isn't this illegal Bernard?"

"Fuck no – it's publishing!"

Jackson closed his eyes and saw blood red red red as death. "I want to see their revisions first."

"Fine." Bernard leaned back in his chair and scratched. He belched and poured himself a cup of mineral water – Vichy water in fact.

Jackson waited for the revisions and looked at the FAX – nine pages single spaced – in horror. "I can't do this Bernie."

"Jack, listen to me. If we sign a contract by Thursday midnight, you can get shares in Rockford House. Then you can bitch and moan about the book. Sell me your shares - I have a buyer. If the deal goes sour, you're out nothing and we can shop the book to another publisher. To be honest Jack, I don't think it will sell, it doesn't fit your image. But, if it does sell, you will have the advance from Rockford, the money from me, and a new contract for two books, one of them a potboiler, the other *The Honest Man*. Understand?"

"Okay Bernie. Play it that way. I'll be at the Hotel Olcott if you need me."

"You and Sara over?"

"I guess fuck bitch yes."

"You screwing the kid, Maggie?"

"Yeah."

"Have her get a HIV test, Jack. Talk to you tomorrow kiddo with good news."

TWENTY SIX

Nelson Rockford agreed to all of the requests of Bernard Crawford, and offered a contract for three books, one a sequel to *Backstabbers!*, one a new novel and the third *The Honest Man*. Crawford agreed that they could hold off on the publishing of *The Honest Man* by one year if Nelson agreed to a stock trade in lieu of advance. The royalty rate for the three books went up over sales of 100,000 copies (Nelson couldn't see the sequel failing to achieve that but was nervous about the other two books. Al Fredericks thought it was okay though – assuming the baseline royalty rate was kept the same under 100,000 units.) Nelson also agreed to Sara editing the three books as chief editor, an unusual request from Jackson but one he insisted on. Nelson figured he would tell her after Friday night.

The deal was closed by Rockford and Crawford at 1:00 Wednesday during a expensive lunch at the Four Seasons. Bernie wondered if he could get Jackson to agree to everything by Thursday night and sign the contract. One way to find out ...

"Jack, it's Bernie. Can you meet me for a drink at Yoshihara Towers?" Yoshihara had bought the ornate building from Donald Trump in a business decision more orientated by Yoshi's sense of personal irony than anything else. New kid on the block? Bullshit, he had saved Trump's neck when everyone else had turned away from him.

After his fifth scotch Jack was willing to sign anything, not even bothering with the finer details. He would be rich, his beloved book would come out – although when was not specified in the contract – a point Crawford didn't point out to Jackson – and he could start his next novel – although it was the sequel to *Backstabbers!* – another point not emphasized by Bernie.

Jackson left the Yoshihara Towers and Bernard Crawford called up to the penthouse to Yoshi Yoshihara. "It's done Yoshi. You just became the major stockholder in Rockford House. Fifty-one percent of the stock offering. Happy?"

"Happy happy happy." Yoshi crooned. "Now we just sit and wait a day or two ... "

Bernie didn't like the sound of that but he had his commission and didn't really care too much about damage control.

TWENTY SEVEN

Jackson threw up on his shoes and stared at the streets of New York, lined with so much garbage like his personal life. Like the garbage his problems were man-made. He had been treated not as an artist but as an commodity, a thing to be bought and sold. He wondered what to do and thought of killing himself. It was not an idle thought or an irrational one - death fed his dreams and deepest fears like a siren out at sea calling him to his doom. 'Red red red' she calls, crying out his secret name. Her face was a mixture of Millie and Sara's, a thing with two heads and one giant all consuming mouth that lied to him.

But suicide wasn't an option, he had a book coming and Maggie was still with him. Maybe something would work out there, some completeness would emerge from being with her.

He hailed a cab, went uptown to the Hotel Olcott and woke Maggie up. "It's over kid. We head back to Los Angeles tomorrow."

"Don't you want to go to the party at Nelson's?" She asked, mascara lining her eyes like a raccoon, a badge of color that distracted Jackson from staring into her eyes.

"No. I want to go home."

"Can I go to the party alone and meet you in Los

Angeles on Sunday?"

"Sure." Jackson was willing to give her that. What was she willing to give? "Give me a blow job?"

It was futile though - Jack had been screwed totally and was out of any passion or interest. After twenty minutes Maggie applied some lip gloss to herself, tucked Jackson into bed, and watched a rerun of *Star Trek*. Some things were better than sex.

TWENTY EIGHT

The announcement that Rockford House had signed Jackson Evans to a three book contract, including the sequel to *Backstabbers!*, broke at nine in the morning Friday. The stock offering went up over the course of the day and the stock closed at $45.75 a share. On Saturday morning Nelson Rockford called Bernard Crawford up and advised him he was voiding the contract due to Jackson's medical and drinking problems. Bernie hemmed and hawed but agreed that the advance would be returned. Yoshi Yoshihara had already sold back his entire interest in Rockford House at the close of Friday, on the inside information from Nelson that he was going to drop Jackson Evans. Yoshihara was ahead two million dollars; Nelson had regained control of his publishing house, and Jackson Evans was out of a publishing deal. This left him broke on paper, with his investments from the previous two books having been wasted over the last six months on trips and the buying of the house in California. It was Jackson's only remaining asset, except for future royalties, and most of the sales life of his two books was over with the rough cut of *Backstabbers!* having been screened the week before to a hostile audience. Now Jackson had to start again, regain his perspective, and his career.

And his agent. Bernard Crawford dropped him Monday morning. Jack sat in his house and took a long sip of Scotch. The drink warmed him, and made a good breakfast. "Bitch shit fuck," he Touretted in the empty air. Maggie hadn't returned from New York and her telegram of resignation was dropped on the floor, like a loose sock or a forgotten child's toy.

Jack wondered if there was anything left in his life that belonged to him, other than his life itself. He picked up a steak knife and touched it lightly to his wrist, seeing red red red as blood in his mind, hearing the sound of dripping blood and wondering if this time he was really cracking up. He stood up, and threw the knife to the floor.

"Where are those fucking mermaids when I need them," he asked the air. He picked up the knife and held it to his wrist and cut. Then he began to scream, quietly at first then with more force. He couldn't stop – wouldn't stop – and when the police showed up twenty minutes later, he was drenched in blood from the self inflicted cuts on his arms.

Publishing sucks.

TWENTY NINE

It was two days later.

"Dr. Collins will see you now, Mr. Evans." Nurse Susanne Smith said quietly to the heavily medicated Jackson. He stood up unsteadily, then fell back in his wheel chair. Susanne sighed – she wouldn't be getting an autographed copy of *Backstabbers!* today – and motioned to the dozing attendant, Jesse. Jesse came over to Jackson and began wheeling him into the neurologist's office.

What a long strange trip it's been, thought Jackson, flashing onto a line from a Grateful Dead song. Betrayal, rape, and attempted suicide. Almost more fun to live life than to write it – fuck shit Nazis in pink wet pant suits like Godzilla's on speed ... Jackson dozed off and Jesse yawned.

Dr. Collins greeted Jackson sadly, wondering what had thrown him over the edge so violently. Dr. Collins glanced through his notes and noticed that Jackson had slashed his wrists not lengthwise, the normal suicide approach, but had nicked himself cross sectionally from the tips of his fingers to his elbow on his left hand, drawing blood but not cutting deep. Then he had stabbed the knife

89

into his right palm, leaving a deep incision. Weird, thought Dr. Collins, the pathology isn't right for suicide. But what else could it have been-self torture or self mutilation?

Dr. Collins looked at Jackson and Jackson looked back dully. Thousand yard stare, thought Dr. Collins, the marine on the move. Dr. Collins waved the attendant out of the room and the door shut firmly, like a trim bookend on Jackson's tiny shelf of bestsellers. Jackson started at the sound and held his left bandaged hand in his right, clutching it almost like a talisman, stroking the fingers alternately with deep breaths.

"What happened Jackson? Did you try to kill yourself?"

Jackson looked blankly at Dr. Collins and began to cry. "It hurts."

"The cuts?"

"No, the itching, the tingling, the sensations in my body. I wanted to dull the pain by distracting my feelings, but I must have misjudged what I was doing, didn't focus the lens through time correctly ... "

Dr. Collins thought about what he had discussed with Jackson earlier that year. "Do you mean Sensory Tourette symptoms, a painful sensation that must be fulfilled correctly before you can finish a tic?"

"Fuck shit. Yeah. It still bothers me though, mud puppies, even with all of the drugs you pumped me full of. Red red red. How long will I be here?"

That was sudden – shot out of left field, Dr. Collins thought. His mind is really racing now, jumping from thought to thought. "You have to stay as an inpatient for seventy-two hours for observation, then we'll decide what to do with you in terms of further treatment. I'd like you to voluntarily commit yourself for three weeks while we stabilize your medications."

"Okay." Jackson stood up suddenly, then fell back into the wheelchair, his back arching violently. He landed on his left bandaged hand and screamed. The attendant burst into the room, eagerly anticipating an attack on the doctor. Jackson was wheeled away for another injection of Thorazine, and Dr. Collins wondered what to do with a patient whose chief mental illness was his biological brain disorder.

THIRTY

Over the next few days the inpatient center at the small Woodland Hills Hospital where Dr. Collins had a neuropsychiatry ward ricocheted over the fact that a world famous writer was committed there for psychiatric observation. Jackson was secluded from the media attention, although People magazine ran another piece on him and Entertainment Tonight actually ran a piece on a writer over the age of twenty-five other than Norman Mailer, whose problems were chiefly marital not mental. Jackson kept to himself the first week, heavily medicated and healing from his injuries. He dozed often, not noticing much in the way of other people or things, ignoring the television in the wardroom where most of the patients worshiped in the afternoons and early evenings. One evening during reruns of *Alf* he developed an echo of the alien's cry "Aw Willie!"

It lasted for three days and after that he stopped even socializing on that level. He was unresponsive to group therapy or individual analysis, to the point that his therapist, Linda Macatee, suggested to Dr. Collins that she be taken off the case.

"He's so distrustful of people that I almost wonder if he would be better off left asleep until he was ready to wake up. All he can respond to when we talk is to look down my blouse occasionally, then look away embarrassed."

"That's a good sign Linda."

"Why?"

"Impotency has been a problem of his for the last several years. If he's starting to get interested in sex again ..."

"It's not sex, it's just looking."

"He's got to start somewhere again." Dr. Collins cracked his knuckles and thought to himself what to do for Jackson. He didn't want to have to change therapists for Jackson, but after ten days he was still in the same dazed shell shocked state he had been brought in with. Perhaps there was another answer, another therapeutic modality ...

Dr. Macatee said brightly, "Do you think a sex surrogate would be in order when he's ready to deal with people again?"

Dr. Collins smiled. "Good thought. Do you have one in mind?"

"Goodness no, I never used one for a patient before. I just thought ... "

Dr. Collins picked up his phone. "I know just the person. Jillian Kerridge. She's a playwright, not too attractive, but full of the intellectual tensions that Jackson enjoys."

"Shouldn't she be attractive? I mean, if he's going to

sleep with her ... ?"

"I'm not going to indulge his fantasies Linda. He needs to work, not play. Besides, if Jillian can't get a rise out if him - wrong choice of words that - if Jillian can't rouse him out of his stupor then nobody can."

Jillian answered and Dr. Collins described the situation to her, Dr. Macatee listening in, in sinful fascination. The new science of sex surrogates seemed sick to her, but everybody was having such good results with them these days. Besides, in these days of AIDS and Herpes lesions the thought that professionals would really lay it on the line with their patients intrigued her. But she by far preferred her vibrator.

THIRTY ONE

Dr. Macatee sat back and watched Jackson lie on the couch. He was more responsive today, his need for sedatives reduced over the last week. He glanced at her and for a moment their eyes met, then Jackson twitched and looked away, flushing.

"Jackson, I want to talk to you about bringing in another ... therapist to work with you."

"Why?" He asked dully.

"Because she has skills I don't have."

"Bitch."

"Pardon? Oh, that was a tic. Anyway, Dr. Collins and I would like you to see a sex surrogate."

Jackson arched his back and grunted. "A what?"

"A sex surrogate. She's a therapist who uses sexual touching as a treatment modality."

"Does that mean I have to fuck her?"

Dr. Macatee flinched. "No need to be blunt Jackson. But essentially, from what I understand about surrogates, their work includes intercourse."

"I'm not interested."

"Why not?"

"I'm impotent for Christ's sake! Don't you know what that means? I can't get it up. Jesus, use your brain." Jackson was roaring at her. Dr. Macatee felt a little frightened but also delighted - they had hit on a central issue here and the idea of a sex surrogate was now making more sense to her.

"It's because of your impotency that we want you to see the surrogate. We think that your medication alone isn't the cause of your sexual problems."

"Oh really."

"You masturbate almost every night in your room Mr Evans."

"You must love to watch."

"You're not exactly subtle and the nurse has walked in on you several times. So your inability to achieve an erection isn't an issue. It's an issue of relationships, and your lack of ability to have fulfilling ones."

"So you think if I pay someone to fuck me I'll be happy? I could just go to a massage parlor and save everybody a hassle."

"Jack, this isn't sex for money. It's therapy."

"Oh, I see. Bad sex for money."

"Cute. No really, this is a recognized treatment in cases

such as yours. Dr. Collins will supervise, he has more experience with these things than I. Will you think about it?"

"Okay." Jackson glanced at Dr. Macatee's legs and she pulled her skirt down. She blushed. I really have to get better with these kinds of sessions, she thought, I'll ask my therapist about it next week.

"This is your first off hospital grounds pass, Jackson. I want you to promise me something." Dr. Collins asked.

"I won't go on a binge. I haven't had a drink in three weeks and frankly the Prozac you got me on is making me nauseous."

Dr. Collins smiled. "Good. We understand each other. You're due back at five, but you can have a little leeway after your session with Jillian if you need it."

"Thanks, Dr. Collins."

"Tim."

Jackson smiled for the first time in weeks, and held his still healing hand out to Dr. Tim Collins. "Tim. Am I actually going to fuck this woman?"

"Maybe. It depends on the course of your therapy and whether you can handle the intimacy of it. This is therapy – not a massage parlor. Your demands are not the main ones here."

Jackson shrugged. "Aw Willie, buy popcorn! There goes the weasel – God, I have to stop watching television while my echolalia is this bad."

Tim laughed. "It could be worse – the ward could get cable!"

"Or show the film of *Backstabbers!*"

THIRTY TWO

Jillian lived and worked in a tiny Spanish style bunga-low in Van Nuys. Jackson arrived on time, got out of his car, walked to the door, went back to his car and started the motor. He stopped the motor, lit his pipe and drew in. It felt good after three weeks of not smoking and he thought vaguely of a drink, but he had promised Dr. Collins – Tim. He went back to the door and rang the bell.

Jillian was about thirty (Oh God another younger woman) and had her hair pulled back in a long red ponytail. She smiled at Jackson and waved him into the living room. There was a futon made up on the floor, a pile of towels, a bottle of massage oil and a tiny bronze figure of Buddha. On the walls were Japanese prints of Mount Fuji by Hiroshige, and on top of the piano a small vase of dried flowers. Jackson felt at peace here.

"I've never worked with a famous, or is it infamous, writer before, Mr. Evans ..."

"Jack is what my close friends call me."

"You see me as a close friend? That's odd, considering we've just met." Jillian had a soft voice tinged with humor.

Jackson warmed to her immediately. She motioned him to sit on the couch. She sat next to him.

"In every man's life there comes a time when you have to let down the defenses and admit in friends. My time came three weeks ago when I tried to kill myself. If I want to fucking choose you as a friend I think I have that right. At sixty dollars a hour I demand it."

Jillian turned her lip up in a grimace. "Well, what else do you demand? Should I strip and spread 'em now or do you want a blow job first?" Her voice had changed into a growl now.

Jackson stopped twitching his neck, confused by her response. What the Hell was going on here? The banter had been almost fun at first but now it seemed like real life. "I want to talk for while. That's all. If you think making love is in order, well, I haven't had an erection in a month. Good luck."

"Look Jack, I won't play rough with you. I can tell you like to put on a front at times and if we can't get beyond that we can't work together at all. I'm sorry about what happened to you. But this is therapy and we need to set up some ground rules before we become friends. Okay?"

"Okay. What are they?"

"I call all the shots about sexual relations."

Jackson stood up and paced. "Control game?"

"No, woman's right to choose. I'm not attracted to you Jack, I may never be with your bad attitude. But if we have sexual relations, I want the right to say no without you treating me like shit."

"Okay." Jackson sat down again, next to Jillian, but not too close. She moved towards him and laid a hand on his leg. He shuddered slightly from the contact.

"Be calm dear. There will be no condomless penetration."

"Of course." Jesus this was sounding clinical. She sounded like a textbook on sex in the 1990's. No, she sounded like Sara. Whoa.

"You can't make comments about my weight, and during my period I demand back rubs."

Jackson grinned. "This is more like it, but your weight seems fine bitch."

Jillian crossed her eyes oddly at Jackson and he laughed. "Was that one of your famous tics?"

"You bet."

"I don't like them. They bother me. I feel very uncomfortable with people who are obviously disabled and your twitching and swearing are going to bother me."

Jackson started to stand up but Jillian held his hand. He stayed and she said quietly, "this is supposed to be analogous to a real relationship. Surely other woman have been bothered by your Tourette syndrome symptoms before?"

"Yes, but fuck not so bluntly."

"Our time together is short. Usually ten sessions. I have to be very up front and I want you to be as well. How do you feel about being here?"

"Sick."

Jillian nodded. "In one sense you are. But not in the sense you're thinking of. You're not crazy, you're not mentally ill. I don't work with those kind of clients. But you're impotent. I can help you with that." Jillian lowered her voice and touched Jackson's arm. "Please let me help you with that?"

"Okay. What do we do?" Jackson was feeling terrorized and had no idea how to unwind. Was she going to take her clothes off, was he going to be asked to do something sexual after ten minutes of conversation? It was embarrassing, and Jackson's neck began to jerk up and down in sequences of five.

"Relax. Take off your shoes." Jillian stood up and headed into the kitchen. Jackson heard the water tap running. He wondered what to do, then slid off his sandals. He looked at the artwork and wondered if Jillian played piano. He wanted to touch middle C to see if it was in tune. He realized he was obsessing and tried to concentrate on the here and now. A car honked outside and Jackson wondered what key the horn was in. He felt disturbed.

Jillian came back and kneeled in front of Jackson with a wash bucket full of water. "I'm going to slowly wash your feet. I want you to pay full attention to what it feels like - how you feel. Then if you're willing to, you're going to wash mine."

"What does this have to do with sex?"

"Trust. Compassion. Building a relationship. Stuff like that."

Jackson slid his feet into the luke warm water and sighed. "About that blow job ... "

"Out of the question. Today."

Jackson closed his eyes and for the first time in months just felt. He didn't think about his books, or Sara, or the red red red lurking just at the corner of his left eye begging him to twitch. Instead he breathed deeply and let Jillian wash his feet. It was pleasurable and intimate and Jackson wasn't sure he liked it. But he felt relaxed. The music in his head faded, the outside noise ceased to penetrate the peace of Jillian's living room. Jackson was aware of the temperature of the water, her hands rubbing the bottom of his feet, the wetness of the water and how cool the air seemed in contrast as his feet slid in and out of the water.

Jackson washed Jillian's feet with extra attention

drawing her toes apart and bathing them in the healing epsom salted waters of the bucket. She sighed deeply and murmured at one point, "slower." Jackson started to laugh - the sexual analogy amusing him, then he realized it wasn't an analogy at all, but the real thing. He took his time and when he was done, bent down, lifted her feet and kissed her right big toe.

Jillian smiled. "Good work for today Jack."

Jackson paid her, and headed out to his car feeling more complete than he had in a long time. It wasn't sexual - it wasn't about arousal or orgasms or the purring sound a woman makes when you touch her the right way, but it was the deep satisfaction of making love on an intimate level that Jackson had lost somewhere in the violence of the last few years.

THIRTY THREE

At the next week's session they just talked, mostly about Jackson's relationships with women, particular Millie and Sara. Jillian was intrigued to hear that Jackson hadn't achieved an orgasm during intercourse since his divorce.

"You don't find that odd?" She asked.

"Well, intercourse has always been difficult for me. Something about totally letting go, unwinding to the state where I can enjoy it ... "

"But you had intercourse with Millie?"

"I fucked her."

"Did you enjoy it?"

Jackson was thrown by the question. Enjoy it? "Well, to be honest I did it because I felt she wanted it. I liked to hold her, to kiss her, to pet her, to go down on her, but the act, the fucking always seemed strained. I was usually drunk when it worked out and I never liked it as much as she did. I think the reason she fucked Henry was because he could give her something I couldn't."

"Could she achieve orgasm without ... fucking?"

"Oh yeah, she came all the time." Jackson stopped for a moment and thought about it. "At least I think she did. She claimed she did, but she was such a bitch at times ... "

"Did she like it as much as intercourse or are you just guessing?"

"I think she liked fucking the best. Although we didn't do it for two years or so, and when we did, it was because she insisted. I really wasn't ready."

"What was your first time like?"

"Awful. I didn't come."

"You didn't come? At all? Had you before with Millie?"

"Yes."

"So the problem isn't impotency, it's intercourse. You don't like it."

Jillian looked at Jackson and he blinked. She seemed to be on to something here. "But doesn't everybody like fucking? Is there something wrong with me that I don't like it?"

"No, there's nothing wrong with you. Different people get sexual pleasure from different things. You like oral sex, mutual masturbation, kissing. I like intercourse. It's just a different taste, like red wine versus white. The outcome is the same, orgasm. You just get to it in a different way. When you had intercourse with Sara ... "

"We never did."

Jillian blinked. "Not once?"

"We tried it a few times but she would get so uptight and I would lose my erection. It seemed like she enjoyed the same things I did, so we stopped trying after awhile."

"Did she want to have intercourse with you?"

"I don't know."

"This secretary ... "

"Maggie. That bitch."

"You had intercourse with her?"

"Once. I practically raped her."

"Did you come?"

"Yes."

"Did you like it?"

"God no. It was awful, I said I raped her."

"Was that your intent, did that aspect give you pleasure?"

"No."

"What did? The intercourse?"

"I guess. It was the spontaneity of it, the lack of red red red ..."

"Red red red?" Jillian was thrown by that, it was the first time Jackson had referred to his obsession.

"The intrusive colors and sounds I hear and see. I didn't have them that morning. I just felt horny and she ... was there. So I fucked her."

"Did she like it?"

"Yes."

"Did you have intercourse again with her?"

"We tried, but I always was soft. Look, this is getting pretty painful, this conversation."

Jillian moved closer to Jackson and put her arms

around his shoulders. He was starting to weep. She hugged him for a long moment. "Would you like to have intercourse with me at some point?"

"I don't know. Maybe."

"Jack, I think I can help you learn ways to relax during sex. Whether you'll like it is up to you. I think you are fully capable of achieving good healthy orgasms through intercourse. I know you are. You just have some problems getting to it – you're blocked by your Tourette syndrome medications and your past history. You expect to fail so you do. Self-fulfilling prophecy is the term we use. Do you understand what I'm saying?"

Jackson nodded, breathing in the fragrance of Jillian and her long red hair. "I think so."

Jillian handed Jackson a book. He glanced at it. It was *Cannery Row* by John Steinbeck. "One of my favorites. I think the reason I love Monterey so much is because of this book."

Jillian tapped the book. "Learn the life style in this. Don't worry about past events, cause and effect situations. Just live now, in the present. It will work itself out and you'll be the happier for it." Jackson kissed the top of her head and she smiled at him.

"Enough for today. What about a back rub?"

"I'd love one." Jackson said.

Jillian smiled. "I meant for me!" She grinned and pushed him onto the futon. "Okay, but you owe me one next week." She began to unbutton his shirt and he tensed. She stopped. "I can rub your back with your shirt on but it won't feel as nice." Jackson pulled his shirt off and nodded.

Jackson lay on the futon, shirt off while Jillian kneaded the tension out of his back and shoulders. She dug in deep, causing Jackson to wince once or twice and then suddenly he was crying while she massaged him. It was good.

THIRTY FOUR

Jackson had ignored most of his mail while at the hospital, leaving that to the secretary Sara had hired for him after Maggie left his employ. Sara would forward a letter occasionally from one of his fans, along with a personal note of her own. He read her notes with an irritated feeling – can't she let go, leave me alone?

He also looked forward to knowing that somewhere, someone still cared about him. He had started a corre-spondence with Jason Watkins and his mother Irene in Monterey. They extended an open invitation to him to come visit the Rap Group when he was up to it.

When the day came to go home, to become an outpatient instead of an inpatient, he shared a turkey sandwich with Dr. Collins, who had become a friend. "What should I do now, Tim?"

"Well keep on seeing Dr. Macatee and myself, continue working with Jillian, if you want to ..."

"I want to. I'm learning a lot about myself from her."

"Good. You love Big Sur, that's where you go to renew yourself, isn't it?"

"Monterey, Carmel, Big Sur. Steinbeck country. What about it?"

"Why not plan a trip up there for a weekend? Take your car, your CD player and just get away? Don't drink, don't smoke dope, just unwind. What do you think?"

"Well, I have this invitation to visit the Monterey Tourette Syndrome Rap Group. They meet every month. Maybe I'll go, spend some time seeing how other Touretters live."

"Touretters?" Tim asked, laughing at the word.

"That's what they ... we ... call ourselves."

"I think that's a great idea Jack. But seriously, go with a cool head, don't binge out just because you're out of here."

"I know Tim. You don't have to keep reminding me. I have an AA meeting tonight that I'm looking forward to."

"Good. See you next week?"

"Yes. Thanks Tim. For everything."

Jackson drove home with a sense of deep remorse. Back to his home - back to the trampled life he left behind. Soon he would have to start making some decisions about his life. But first he had a letter to Monterey to write ...

THIRTY FIVE

Irene Watkins answered the door and Jackson was immediately taken with her. She was about his age, with wavy brown hair and dark penetrating eyes that blink blink blinked as much as his own did. Jackson felt that he had finally met a woman who would understand him. The illusion was shattered a moment later when her boyfriend walked up behind her, but the contact, the meeting of somebody else with Tourette syndrome answered an internal loneliness that was a long time being fulfilled.

"Mr. Evans..." She began.

"Jack."

"Irene. Whoa. This is Pablo, my boyfriend. Jason will be back in a few minutes, whoa I sent him to the store. Come in come in."

Jackson sat on the couch, drinking a cup of coffee while Irene told him about the Rap Group that would be meeting that evening. It had a fluctuating membership with anywhere from five to twenty people with Tourette syndrome showing up. Irene also held a group for parents of children with Tourette syndrome but in Jackson's honor just the Touretters would be coming tonight.

"They are all pretty excited. Whoa."

"Indeed. I never met anyone else with Tourette syndrome before, Irene. It seems so strange not to be apologizing or explaining myself to people."

"Even with all of the press you've had?"

"It never stops, bitch shit, the explaining, the looks, the stares from over someone's eyeglasses, the look - look away in a restaurant, the hostile encounter at the bank. Am I going too fast?" Jackson said, laughing.

Irene smiled. "You sound like everyone else at their first encounter. Whoa. Look, here's Jason!"

Jason Watkins stood in the doorway, his lanky frame topped by a head of brown crew cut hair. "You're Jack! Yippie!" Jason leaped into the room, arms akimbo, legs kicking out of control, neck snapping and grunts emerging from his throat. He tried to shake hands with Jackson but ended up hugging him, tears filling his eyes. "Thank you so much for coming here."

Irene grinned. "He's a little impulsive at times. We're

working on that."

"Fuck you mom. I didn't mean that. That was a tic."

"I know. Whoa." Irene twitched her shoulder. Jason cracked up. "Look at mom, she caught that one from me!"

"Caught it?" Jackson asked nervously.

Irene explained. "When you're around other people with Tourette syndrome there's a certain trading of symptoms, a give and take almost. I sometimes will 'borrow' one of Jason's whoa every so often, and he sometimes picks up one of mine."

"Shit. I didn't mean that mom."

"You don't have to apologize every time Jason." Pablo said gently.

"I know what you're feeling though Jason. I used to want to apologize all the time too." Jackson said.

"What do you shit do now?"

"I say 'fuck 'em if they can't take a joke' Sorry Irene."

The four of them laughed and Irene said after they quieted down, "I hope you haven't booked a hotel room or anything in town."

"Well, not yet. I usually stay in Big Sur at Ventana."

"One of our members, Carrie Jefferson, usually puts people from out of town up at her place. She lives south of the Carmel Highlands. She insisted I make the offer. She's very nice."

"She has great tics," Jason offered.

"Pretty too," Pablo added.

"Don't you go setting up Jackson you two. I'm sure he has a girlfriend in Los Angeles. Whoa. Don't you Jack?"

"Well, no. At least not one with great tics." Jack laughed nervously — they were joking, right? "You're joking, right?"

Irene grinned. "Don't worry Jack, these two just like to

107

play matchmaker. Whoa."

"Whoa indeed." Jason laughed at Jackson and began to ask him questions about his writing, how much he wrote a day, if he read when he was writing, who his favorite writers were, what his next book was going to be about. Jackson relaxed and just enjoyed the company, all Touretting away except for Pablo who listened intently and occasionally asked a question. When dinner time came they sent out for pizza and continued getting to know each other.

THIRTY SIX

Invisible insects assail his skin.
He begins to fidget and twitch.
He knows what he's done is a sin.
And he shouts out 'bitch'.

Tensions increase – he starts to yell.
The white coats are at the hospital waitin'.
He knows that he is going straight to hell.
For what he does comes from Satan.

Don't cry Jason, hold on tight,
This too will pass, this lonely night,
Morning will come with new blessings,
Instead of fear there will be guessing,
That God loves children with Tourette,
And what they now suffer, they will soon forget.

THIRTY SEVEN

The meeting room at the local community college was semi full by the time Jackson arrived. The room was LOUD – people grunting, vocalizing, swearing, banging chairs, hitting themselves. Jackson started to back out of the room warily but was stopped by a firm hand. He glanced behind him and saw a young woman with an outstanding length of long whitish blond hair down to her waist. Her eyes were a whitish shade of blue, and her skin was etched delicately with thin blue veins. She smiled at Jackson, while staring at his crotch. "Hi. You're new here. Wanta fuck?"

"Pardon?" Jackson asked, wondering if his fly was undone.

"One of my tics. Carrie Jefferson." She held out her hand to him.

"Jackson Evans." He replied, shaking it.

"Oh wow! You're the writer. Fuck me! Did Irene give you my invitation, wanta suck me off?"

"Yes, Irene did give me your invitation bitch. Are you sure it wouldn't be a bother?"

"In my bed! No, not at all." She smiled and Jackson was lost in her eyes which reminded him of the tint of the dawn tinged ocean at Monterey. "I hear you like Big Sur. I work down there."

"What do you do Carrie?"

"Fuck horses. I'm a masseuse at the Esalen Institute four days a week, and I also conduct the local chamber orchestra in the Sur."

"That's great. You're a fuck musician?"

"Flute. Great for the embouchure, and it teaches you how to breathe correctly. Do you play?"

"I play drums."

Irene walked up to them, head shaking to the right. "Whoa. I see you two have already met."

"I'm going to fuck him Irene."

Irene grinned. "Isn't she great, Jack? I knew you two would hit it off."

"Can I talk to you a minute, Irene?" Jack asked nervously. Carrie pinched him on the behind and walked to a chair. "Is she coming on to me or are those her regular tics?"

Irene started to laugh, then realized Jackson was serious. "Nope, sorry to disappoint you Jack, but that's just her whoa Tourette."

"It's ... interesting. I've never seen it so severe before. Does she have physical tics too?"

"Real bad sometimes but she's relaxed here. She'll tell you about her tics if you ask."

Right, Jackson thought. I bet there's nothing she wouldn't talk about. Or am I assuming too much from her coprolalia? I know so little about this damn disorder. I guess I'm in the right place to start my education.

The meeting lasted over three hours. Irene introduced Jackson to the crowd and they cheered as he spoke nervously to them. "I've never met anyone else with Tourette syn-

drome before today and I'm a little scared by you all. I guess
you know I've had some problems recently. I'm here
tonight trying to find out how you're all coping and whether
I can learn anything from you that will help me put my life
back together."

Jack sat down, next to Irene and Pablo. A young man,
with silver framed eyeglasses and a tendency to rock back
and forth in his chair in units of three raised his hand. "I
guess what you are talking about is suicide despair death
wishes."

"Yeah." Jack responded, stunned by the man's blunt-
ness.

"We all go through that sometimes. It's part of being
disabled, different in this fascistic culture. I was in Norway
last year and it really shook me up - no one stared, nobody
laughed at my tics. They were civilized, unlike this country
run by mad dogs of the right."

"Mark's right," a middle aged woman with a throat
clearing sound added. "I go to the bank, same bank I've
been going to for ten years and there are times when the
guard still looks at me like he wants to blow me away for
being so noisy."

"Or just twitching," another man added. "You would
think that people would get used to it but except for friends
they don't. They always look at you like you're a criminal
- the bad guy. I work at a temp agency, doing data entry. I'm
good at what I do, but no one has ever offered me a full time
position. I can't afford health insurance on my own so I do
without. It makes me angry."

"And sad." Carrie offered. "You see Jackson, not all of
the issues, fuck me whore me, are as serious as suicide. But
they all hurt people. Where I work it takes me thirty minutes
to drive there, and during that drive I'm screaming my

111

words and twitching away. Then at work I hold it in while I'm with a client. Then I take a break, get into a hot spring and twitch away for a few minutes. It helps, letting it out in intense bursts like that."

"But you can't always live your life that way, Carrie." Mark said angrily. "Sometimes you're in the office eight to ten hours at a time and if you keep it in you explode - your tics come pouring out of you so fast you can't function sometimes. Then what? How do you explain that to your boss?"

"Well you can't sometimes," Jackson offered. "But does your boss know you have Tourette?"

"It doesn't matter," Mark snapped back hostilely. "You think that because you're rich you got it made, work at home, support the ruling classes. But it's different when you work in an office."

"Hey man, fuck, I worked in a office until five months ago. Not my own office either, we were a little company. Bitch. There were three of us in one medium sized room, more like a cell, all of us on the phone trying to push records to the press, to radio, and to buyers. My noises interfered a lot at times. But my boss understood, he knew I was good at my job, and the reporters I worked with were under-standing. So don't lay a class trip on me, I've been there too." Jackson felt exhausted by talking about his past but the others in the group seemed to relate to what he was saying. Except for Mark who was perpetually in an angry obsessive haze of conspiracies.

As the group talked and exchanged stories and sug-gestions on coping, Jackson kept on finding his attention diverted by Carrie Jefferson. She was very, well, hip. Very together on the way that she dealt with what appeared to be the most severe case there. She had great 'modes of being', to use one of **Dr.** Macatee's favorite expressions. She seemed incredibly at peace with herself despite the Tourette syndrome symptoms which were constant but, unlike Jackson's invisible obsessions, were markedly apparent at all times. Jackson was aware of another thing too - she was constantly staring at him, then looking away embarrassed by the eye contact when he stared at her. He wondered what the night would bring and felt nervous, wondering if his impotency would be an issue yet again. Then he wondered if he was putting the cart before the horse, fantasizing without a rational basis. Was he so excited about meeting a single woman with Tourette syndrome that he assumed they would end up in bed? Were her tics triggering the images in his mind? He didn't know, nor at the moment did he care. He was having a good time for the first time in months.

THIRTY EIGHT

The meeting didn't end – it kind of trickled off as people slowly left, reluctantly due to the lateness of the hour. Finally Jackson, Irene and Carrie sat together, drinking decaf in little white plastic cups and finishing up the cookies that various people from the group had brought. Irene looked at her watch and laughed. "Whoa! I better get home, Pablo must be worried sick about me. It was great meeting you Jack."

113

Jackson hugged her and she held him tight for a moment. Then she hugged Carrie and left.

"Well, do we go in one car, or do you want to follow me?"

"I'll be glad to drive." Jackson offered.

"Okay. I'm feeling tired and I think my tics are going to explode in another few minutes."

"You didn't let go here?" Jackson asked in confusion. "Everybody else was twitching."

"Yeah, but I feel embarrassed about letting go in a group. Tourette is a very private thing for me. The noises I can't control, but the blinking or the body shakes ... I don't let a lot of people see that. I hope you don't mind them."

"I feel honored that you feel comfortable enough with me to show them."

"Show you my tits too fuck face." Carrie laughed. "Jesus! This disorder is weird, you know?"

Jackson grinned. "Yeah, I know. Let's go."

The drive down Route 1 to Carmel was quiet. Carrie twitched at times but it was nothing like the explosion that she had warned Jackson about. Her vocalizations though were constant – an endless stream of sexual remarks, grunts and at times laughter. Jackson didn't talk, just drove, his mind honing in on the road he loved so much. His thoughts were far away from Carrie for the moment. He remembered the first time Millie had taken him camping in the mountains here, how she burned dinner and they ended up eating in the Big Sur Lodge. Life was easier then.

As they passed Carmel and she gave him directions, she leaned against him on a curve and he put his arm around her. She let him keep it there and snuggled up to him in the car. Jackson was pleased but still unsure of how to let things develop. Should he kiss her? Should he let her make the first

114

move? Did it matter at all, they were so much in tune at this moment ...

When they got to Carrie's little cabin Jackson stopped the car and held her for a moment. She sighed. "Oh Jackson, fuck me."

Jackson laughed. "Was that a proposition or a tic?"

Carrie moved away, startled. "That was a tic! I barely know you."

Jackson felt like an idiot. "I'm sorry Carrie, I thought ..."

"Besides," Carrie continued angrily, "I don't sleep with people with Tourette syndrome. If I get involved with someone fuck me again I want someone with clean genes, not some damn neurological disorder!"

"Christ Carrie, I didn't mean to insult you. It's just the way you were looking at me during the meeting and us holding each other on the drive ... "

"Oh shit, I never met anyone famous before. The drive was nice but it doesn't mean I want to fuck you yes fuck me."

They went into the cabin, Jackson carrying in his overnight bags. Carrie pointed to the couch and they made the bed up in silence except for their tics. Jackson apologized again and Carrie laughed. "You're not the first person to make that mistake Jack. Don't be in a sweat about it. I like you, you like me, let's leave it at that, okay?"

"Okay."

Carrie walked over to Jackson and kissed him lightly on the cheek. He held her but she pulled away after a second. "Good night."

Jackson lay awake for a long time and thought about the encounter. He ended up laughing himself to sleep. There was no other response that made sense to him.

THIRTY NINE

When Jackson got home from Monterey he found a series of strange messages on his answering machine. Besides the usual calls from Millie and a few friends in the music world, there were six calls from Bernie Crawford and even a call from Nelson Rockford. He hadn't heard from either of these men since his return from New York and his breakdown. Why would they call him now?

The phone rang as he was pondering this. "Hello?"

"Jackson? Thank God you're back. It's Bernie. How ya doing baby?"

"What the fuck do you want?" Jackson said angrily.

"Van Beest wants to buy the rights to *Lucia*. He plans on directing and he wants you to write the screenplay. Things move fast in Hollywood - another two days he would have passed on this and done that new Vanessa Redgrave project."

Rik Van Beest was the hottest new property in Hollywood. Winner of the Cannes film festival two years running for best picture, he had moved to Los Angeles and had been courted by three studios. After settling on a production deal with Spielberg for five pictures, he had

116

returned to Holland to play for six weeks with his jazz trio. He was an enfant terrible, and Jackson loved his work. But *Lucia*? As a movie? Well, first things first.

"You don't represent me anymore Bernie. Did you tell Van Beest that?"

"Well, not exactly. But there's more. If this movie happens Rockford House could release the book overseas and do a paperback marketing tie in. You know they're doing their own paperbacks now? Anyway, Nelson has been hounding me over this. He'll do anything to keep you happy."

"Because I own the film rights?" Jackson asked, suddenly figuring out the game.

"Exactly."

Jackson laughed. "Well, I'm keeping them. This book isn't for sale." He hung up, still laughing and looked at his watch. Ten seconds later the phone rang again. Jackson let his machine answer it. It was Bernie, huffing and puffing in anxiety. Jackson finally picked up, chuckling. "Okay Bernie, I'll bite. But there's a few contingencies ... "

"Shoot."

"I want my book out by next year."

"*Lucia* will be out in paperback at the same time as the movie. Say, ten months from now."

"Not that book. *The Honest Man*."

"Oh God." Bernie thought for a moment. "You have a price?"

"I'll let you work it out, but this time there's no commission for you on it. You do the film for ten percent, the paperback deal for ten percent. *The Honest Man* you do for free, to make up for the damage you caused last time around."

Bernie coughed, grunted, swore. "You got a deal Jack

117

baby."

"I want a FAX of a deal memo in twenty minutes or I'm going to call ICM or William Morris."

"Gotch ya. Bye." Bernie hung up. Jackson grinned and felt the old familiar buzz working again. But this time he was in control and held all the cards. The phone rang again. It was Nelson Rockford.

"Jack, look, have you heard from Bernard Crawford?"

"No. I've been out of town, just got back, haven't touched my machine ... "

"Look, Jack, I know you probably bear me some ill will, some hard feelings. I want to make it up to you. I know you're hurting for cash. How about I buy all rights to *Lucia* for two hundred thousand dollars?"

"Gee Nelson, I'm touched. I could really use the money. This is great. You're a real doll." Jackson paused. "Has Rik Van Beest ever read the book?"

Nelson paused in mid sentence. "Van Beest? What's he got to do with this?"

"Oh shit Nelson, you're trying to fuck me over again. I just talked to Bernie. You got the book but I got the rights. If there is going to be a film it's my decision. Got me?"

"I'm sorry Jack. I thought this would let you out of a sticky situation, what with your breakdown and all. You've never written a script after all ... "

"I'm willing to learn how. So fuck off Nelson. You'll be getting a call from Bernie in a few minutes. So wait for it. I think you may find it of interest." Jackson hung up and looked at his watch. Ten minutes this time, the phone ringing simultaneously with the FAX machine beeping.

"Jack? It's Nelson. Congratulation on your new book. Al and I have reconsidered releasing it and we want it out by mid year ... "

Jackson smiled. "Good. The advance?"

"We'll still working on it. You have to realize this has been a hard year for publishing ... "

"Three hundred thousand, fifteen percent royalty."

"After sales of ... "

"All sales after royalty is returned. Got me? Or no deal on the film." Jackson hung up again.

The phone rang. "Nelson?"

"No Bernie. We got a deal with Rockford House. They offered three hundred ... "

"I know Bernie. You don't get any of it though. Right?"

"I could get a little more out of them if you were willing to ... "

"I'm not. FAX me a contract and have Van Beest's people call me. I'll be home tonight."

"Right." Bernie paused. "It's good having you back Jackson."

"Fuck you Bernie. I was never gone."

This time Bernie hung up first.

FORTY

Rik Van Beest lived in Beverly Glen Canyon, just a few minutes away from Jackson but a world away from the frantic life of the San Fernando Valley. At Van Beest's request, Jackson drove over for lunch and a discussion of the script of *Lucia*. Van Beest was a large man, blonde, gregarious and mustached. Rik Van Beest greeted him with a hug, kisses on both cheeks and a warm handshake. He is covering all of his bases, Jackson thought.

Inside the expensive rented home, Van Beest introduced him to his family. "This is Katrina, my love." She was a young blonde woman, about twenty five, Jackson guessed. Elegantly dressed, and smiling, she held a small child in one arm, and two more were hiding behind her legs. "And these are the triplets, Miles, Cannonball and Trane."

The triplets were about five, rough faced blonde kids. They grinned and laughed at Jackson's tics and began rough housing around the living room pretending he wasn't there but aware of his every move. Katrina talked to them for a moment in Dutch and they quietly walked out of the room, all three looking abashed. Trane stuck his tongue out at Jackson and Jackson waved good-bye to him.

"I guess jazz is a big part of your life Rik." Jackson ventured.

"It is my life. I make films to pay for the band."

"I heard your first trio album when it came out. I like your playing but it's all over the place, too ..."

"I know, not what do you say here, commercial? As if music could, or should be, commercial. I play what I feel and I don't feel commercial. I feel free or Latin or bop or all those things at once in a frenzy of floating notes. Do you play?"

"I played drums in high school, but after I got kicked out ... I guess you know about my disorder?"

"The Tourette? Of course. My father is a doctor, a psychiatrist, he treats some patients with it in Amsterdam. I have no problem with it. Neither does Katrina." Rik paused, considering his next words. "We love you even more because of it."

Katrina smiled. "My English not very good yet but I like your writing, Jackson. I can't wait to eagerly see your script."

"Yes. Bitch, the script." Jackson said eagerly. "Rik, how do you see this working out?"

Van Beest smiled shyly and started heading Jackson into a small room off the living room. "The music room. We have a drum set. Let's jam for a while and after lunch we'll talk business. Okay, my friend?"

Jackson nodded, bewildered but pleased to be playing with the man whom Jazziz Magazine called the hottest new jazz pianist since Makoto Ozone. Katrina picked up an upright bass and Van Beest sat down at the piano and began playing a slow series of chords. It was an Ellington tune and Jack picked up a set of brushes and began playing lightly underneath Katrina's fluid bass lines. He realized after a moment that she must be a member of Van Beest's trio, her interplay with him was almost psychic, guessing or knowing

121

what chord he was going to play and then responding with the perfect interval or root note. Jackson played a light pattern on the ride cymbal as Van Beest segued into "Satin Doll", beginning with a flurry of notes that left Jackson and Katrina behind for a moment, then laughingly picking up the tune a few bars in. They played for about a hour, all standards, and then in the middle of a phrase Van Beest stopped.

"You're good for an American. Subtle, no over playing. We have a gig at Catalina's next Friday. I haven't hired a drummer yet. Sit in with us?"

Jackson was stunned. "I would be honored. But will the music be ... "

"We're doing standards this year for the triplets. They have to be exposed to their roots. Ellington, Mingus, Davis and Monk. I'll give you the song book before you leave today."

At lunch they discussed music and Van Beest asked a lot of questions about the American jazz scene, of which he was an interested observer. "Now Eliane Elias has got a good thing going, as does little Michel, but they're not American. Do you not produce any new artists here of note?"

"What about Mitch Forman or Kenny Kirkland? Henry Butler or Kei Akagi? We have plenty of new artists, you just don't get to see them because they're working here, either in the studio or in small bands."

"He's right Rik," Katrina noted. "We haven't gone out to see the scene at all since being here. We must have Jackson take us night-clubbing. Will you?"

"I'd love to," Jackson responded, cutting open a pear and smearing brie on it. He wondered when they would get down to business. Katrina excused herself and Jackson turned to Van Beest. "I don't mean to be rude, Rik but about the script?"

"You're so American, so up front. The script is all there, all written."

Jackson flushed. "It's written already? Then why do you need me?"

Rik grinned at Jackson's anxiety, and sipped at a glass of tea. "I mean the book is perfect as a script. You just have to translate your vision into visuals and poetry. It should be easy. It is very American, straight forward, strong story, good female character, a hero, a bad guy, and lots of music. It's all there, Jackson my friend. We will work together on it, I will show you how to write for movies!"

Jackson relaxed. "Deal. Deadline?"

"I want to start filming in five months, after I record the standards album and tour Japan. So you have twelve weeks or so to write the script before I leave and casting begins. Who do you see as Lucia?"

Jackson and Van Beest discussed the film for six hours that day and the next day Jackson reread the novel and started outlining the script based on Van Beest's concept of an American fairy tale.

FORTY ONE

The next day during his session with Jillian, Jackson talked about his meeting with Van Beest and the trip to Monterey. She listened in delight, holding Jackson's hand as he bubbled over enthusiastically about the last week.

"You know Jack, this is the first time I've seen you happy. It's wonderful, you're a lot more attractive." She leaned against him and he cupped her breast with one hand while rubbing her neck with the other. They had progressed to nudity a week before, first exposing their naked selves across the room from each other, then joining hands in the center of the room and lightly touching each other. Today they were holding and stroking each other, the contact not deliberately sexual, but sensual instead. There were no rules today, Jackson realized. If he were to start kissing her she would probably respond in kind. He kissed her lightly on the lips and she kissed him back. "No tongues Jack. Only rule about kissing."

Well, it still felt nice. They kissed and fondled each other for about twenty minutes and then Jackson found himself with an embarrassed erection. He pointed to it and Jillian laughed. "We'll have to do something about that, I guess." She lifted the bottle of massage oil and slowly sprinkled it over his thighs, up his legs and onto his genitals. He shuddered and lay back. She leaned over him and kissed him lightly, then began to stroke him in a light sensitive hand. Jackson came within a minute.

"My God, it usually takes forever. What was different? Did you use some magic oil or something?"

Jillian grinned and reached for a warm towel. "You were relaxed doll. For the first time you weren't nervous about sex - you were just in the moment. How did it feel?"

"It felt great. But I've been relaxed before ... "

"Drunk is different from relaxed. Alcohol makes orgasm more difficult to attain. I bet you could have had intercourse and enjoyed it as much as that today."

Jackson nodded. "That's what you're going to teach me, how to relax? It seems so simple."

"I'm not going to teach you anything. You did the relaxing. I'm just going show you how to attain that feeling when you want it, when you feel the need for it. To be in the moment, to exist in the now. Not to worry about the past and wonder what if ... It is really very simple but it changes so much." Jillian stared at Jackson and watched his face for a long moment. "You know, you haven't twitched in about ten minutes. Is that normal with arousal for you?"

"Oh yes."

"If I were you I'd be getting laid every hour. It's so great seeing you looking ... normal." Jillian stopped and realized that she was being insensitive about his Tourette syndrome symptoms. She put a hand out to Jackson but he stopped her.

"It's okay Jillian. I know you don't like it. But I'm comfortable with it right now. The medication is working, I feel some control in my life, and I've got friends for the first time in a long time."

"The Van Beest's?"

"Yeah. Odd, I never thought I'd become a jazz musician at my age. I can't wait until Friday night. Can you come?"

"It wouldn't be appropriate, Jack."

"But you'll be there?"

Jillian laughed. "With a date!"

Jackson grimaced and then grinned. "Lie back, I want to try this magic oil on you!"

FORTY TWO

Rik opened a beer and offered one to Jackson. He declined and Rik frowned but didn't say anything. They were sitting by the Van Beest's pool, and Katrina was languidly swimming laps. Jackson watched her for a moment and when he looked over at Rik, he smiled.

"She's beautiful, no?"

"Very. How did you meet her?"

"When I was first in film school I did a short film on musicians. I had been playing piano in a night club for tuition, and one night this lovely woman walks in with a guy. They sit in front of me and start arguing. I finally stopped playing and said to them, 'Either listen to the music or get out!' He left, she stayed, we left together. The next day I found out she was a bass player and I filmed her playing. She was perfect, her hands sensitive and warm, her posture at the upright so exquisite! I began playing duets with her and the next year we formed the trio with Tommy Flynn on drums. When Katrina got pregnant I made my first film, and after the triplets were born began writing the script for my second one. Katrina did the music for that one - all arco bass with percussion. She's a total musician. And

126

I love her very much."

Rik stopped talking and waved at Katrina. She smiled back. "What?" She asked from the pool, Trane and Miles splashing around her.

"You're wonderful!"

"Get to work lazy!"

Rik looked at Jackson and asked, "You have a woman?"

"No, not right now. I was involved, but it fell apart a few months ago. There hasn't been anyone since."

"It's lonely, no?"

"Yes."

Katrina walked up to them and dripped water onto Rik. "Don't be lonely Jack. You have Rik and me. You have the triplets."

Jackson smiled. "I know. Thanks."

Cannonball came running out. "Phone Papa."

Rik went inside. Katrina sat down on his chair, and the triplets jumped into the pool. "No deep end." She called to them.

Trane stuck his tongue out. Jackson was beginning to tell the three apart. Trane was the wise guy, Cannonball the scholar, Miles the bright quiet one. Jackson wondered for a moment what it would be like to have a family, children, a wife, a dog even. He became lost inside himself, fighting with the inner demons of his loneliness. Katrina watched him sadly.

"You want kids?"

"Yes." Jackson said.

"Then why no?"

"A lot of reasons. It never seemed like the right time to start a family. Now I think that my disorder is genetic and I couldn't risk passing it on."

Katrina smiled shyly and took Jackson's hand in hers

for a moment. "You turned out okay."

"For an American!" Rik bellowed. He was standing quietly next to them. Jackson felt embarrassed and took his hand away. Rik laughed. "Don't mess with my woman Jack!"

Katrina asked something in Dutch. Rik nodded. "Our visa's have been troubling us. I can stay all year but Katrina and the triplets will have to go back to Holland before Japan. I'm sorry dear."

Katrina nodded. "It will be good to see home again. Miles wants to see Grandma."

"Miles wants to see his pets, I'll bet. You see Jack, you don't just have children, you have their whole damned menagerie as well. I thought when I first met Katrina, me and this woman, we be happy together. Then the triplets came and there were five of us. Then the cat, then the kittens and the birds and the fish and the horse on the farm. It never ends. I'll just buy them all a fucking zoo!"

Rik laughed tensely. Jackson smiled, feeling he was missing something. The way Rik spoke - did he not like having children, or was it the competition for Katrina's love that he resented? Complicated.

Rik dived into the pool and the triplets swarmed around him. He dunked one, then another into the cool blue water. Katrina leaned over to Jackson and said softly, "He likes you Jack. He needs a friend, not just a writer. You stay as long as you want today."

"Thanks Katrina. I like you all too."

Katrina smiled and lay down, pulling on a pair of sunglasses. Jackson took a sip of water and breathed deeply. It was nice here.

FORTY THREE

Friday morning the Los Angeles Times had an interview with Rik Van Beest, the musical prodigy of film. The picture showed him with the triplets seated at his piano. He spoke about his recordings, his concert tours, his two previous movies and his upcoming film of Jackson Evans' *Lucia*. He also said a lot of things about the state of American jazz players that inflamed the local jazz community and led to two sold out shows at his American debut that night at Catalina's jazz club.

As Jackson sat reading the morning newspaper, and drinking the decaf that he kept to most of the time, he saw scenes from the script coming to life before his eyes. The scene where young Lucia is first taught the secrets of love by an older opera star, the moment when she makes her disastrous debut at the Met, her visit to La Scala with Roger. It was so alive to him and the news that Van Beest had hired Placido Domingo as opera consultant to the film, to correct some of the technical mistakes that Jackson had made in the book, was reassuring. Suddenly everything was going the right way. It was about time.

The phone rang. Jackson stopped day dreaming, saw a

flash of red red red and snapped his neck. "Hello?"

"Jackson, it's Sara. Don't hang up, I'm calling on business."

Sara. She had called him weekly since his suicide attempt and he had refused to speak to her. But, all grudges must end, Jackson figured, and he wondered what to say to her.

"Go ahead."

"It's about the two books. Nelson would like to tie the release of *The Honest Man* to coincide with the film and paperback edition of *Lucia*. Given that timetable, would you be interested in some of the editorial thoughts the staff has been having?"

"Not really. I told Nelson no changes. I meant it five months ago and I mean it now."

"A lot has happened in the last five months Jack."

"No shit." Jackson said bitterly.

"Have you read the manuscript recently?" Sara dove in. "It doesn't hold up. It's a good story but very static, flat characters, no resolution at the end of the book. I think it would be a mistake to release it at what could be a time of new success for your writing career. Especially with all of the publicity your ... accident involved. Do you want people thinking that this is all you are capable of? Do you Jack?"

Jackson listened, trying to figure out her game. But why would Sara even give a damn at this point? He suddenly realized that this wasn't a game or a trick, she was serious about the book and as an editor was just doing her job. He sighed. "Okay, I'll reread it. What would the time table be for a new draft?"

"Six months from now. After you finish the script, you can work on it." Sara stopped suddenly and Jackson wondered what she was thinking. "I'm so happy for you

Jack." She said quietly.

"No regrets?" Jackson asked bitterly.

"Plenty of them Jack. I miss you." There, she had said what she wanted to say. Now it was Jack's turn to give a little. Please give me something Jack, she pleaded inside.

"I'll reread it this weekend. Thank you for calling. Bye."

Sara stared at the telephone and tears welled up in her eyes. "Bastard."

FORTY FOUR

The crowd at the club was full of studio musicians, interested jazz fans and the usual contingent of students from the Musicians Institute down the street. Jackson sat backstage with Rik who was smoking a cigarette and drinking cup after cup of strong black coffee. Rik looked up suddenly. "Does the door to this place lock?"

"Yeah, I think so."

"Lock it please." Jackson did so. Rik took a small vial of cocaine out of his jacket pocket and poured several lines on the table. "Join me, my friend?"

"No thanks Rik. I don't handle stimulants very well."

Rik snorted back the coke and smiled tightly. "My viceless friend. No alcohol, no coffee, no cigarettes, no drugs. No women? Are you gay Jack?"

"No. I'm just not seeing anyone right now. It's a long

story."

"Some of my best friends in Holland are gay," Rik said reassuringly. "Jewish too. You Americans are so concerned about these things, who's what and with whom. I find you a woman Jack. That's what you need right now. A girlfriend."

There was a knock at the door. Rik put away the cocaine and wiped off the table with his shirt sleeve. It was Katrina, excited and blushing. "There's such a crowd, Rik! Amazing, aye?"

"No. They know when genius is among them. Time to play?"

"Soon." Katrina looked at Rik closely and started speaking angrily in Dutch. He answered sharply back and she burst into tears. Jackson felt mystified. What was going on here, everything had been going so well, now Rik was acting like a drug fiend and Katrina had turned shrewish. It was good having friends again but they brought new problems just when Jackson had wearied of stress and intensity. All is red, he thought suddenly, red in the key of C. A note sounded in his head and the room spun crimson.

There was another knock at the door and Rik smiled at Jackson. "Now we play."

"Yeah," he said flatly.

Rik patted him on the back. "Go do it friend."

FORTY FIVE

Henry Larkin was six months older than Jack, and had spotted him when they were in band together. After Jack left school, and was banished from the social life of the teenagers in Albany, Henry and Millie were the only two peers he saw. Everyone else was an adult or a relative. Jack hated the isolation but was grateful for Millie and their sexual experimenting, and for Henry and his record collection.

It was Henry who first turned Jack onto jazz. In 1970, when they were both fifteen and listening to the Beatles, the Stones and the first album by Led Zeppelin, Henry rather excitedly brought over a double album by Miles Davis called *Bitches Brew*. It was potent stuff. A swirling rhythm section of drummers, percussionists, two bass players and multiple keyboards played under the muted and amplified trumpet of Miles, the sizzling guitar of John McLaughlin and the reeds of Wayne Shorter and Bennie Maupin. Henry and Jack would listen to it for hours and try to follow along specific instruments as they pulsated in the background. It was a brave experiment in what in another year would be called jazz rock fusion, or simply fusion jazz. Jack would sit in his room, beating out the patterns he heard in the record and singing along with them.

Henry played acoustic bass. He would bring it over sometimes, and Jack would play along on his father's conga drum, left over from teenage years in the beat generation. They would play savage duet's, exploring odd time patterns, styles of soloing and the eternal metric breakdown that Jack heard below the red red red in his mind except when he was making love to Millie or playing drums. Millie would watch the two of them play, noticing that Jack didn't tic when he drummed; she and Henry encouraged him to take up the drum set seriously. But those days seemed over for Jack who knew he would never make it as a professional musician. It was writing he was interested in, even then, and the first short stories to flow from his pen in his large illegible script were fantasies and tales of King Arthur. Later on he started writing about music, trying to capture the rhythms of jazz in words. He must have done something right because for awhile he wrote for *down beat* magazine as a record reviewer and social critic. But that was five years in the future. Right now it was the downbeat and Jack was crazily trying to keep up with Henry and his arrangement of "Giant Steps" for bass. He always had trouble matching Henry's tempo's, but soon he wouldn't have that problem. His ears would retrain themselves and his hands would follow, his chops getting cleaner and faster.

Of course, catching up wasn't the answer. By the time Jack realized that he was living in Los Angeles and working for Dig It Records, listening to the west coast brand of light fusion of the '80's, and sometimes wanting to play again. He kept a practice pad around and at night when things weren't going well, he would practice rolls and timekeeping. After Millie and Henry moved in together the duets, both of them, stopped for good. But the playing - that was the key. Jack lost sight of that in the messiness of the divorce.

FORTY SIX

Rik began "Giant Steps" suddenly and the musicians in the audience applauded the choice. Jackson kept up with the fast tempo of the John Coltrane song by keeping his hi hat and ride cymbal the center of his playing. He would worry about the accents on another song: Right now he needed to provide rhythmic support to the best of his ability. During Katrina's solo he switched to brushes and just sock cymbal, clinking on 2 and 4, beating out ting ting a ling on snare drum with the brushes. After Katrina finished Jackson exploded into a series of four bar trades with Rik, playing rapid snare drum rolls that hid his less then perfect technique. But the time was there.

After the set they went back to the dressing room where Rik had another three lines of coke and Katrina yelled at him in Dutch again. People began coming backstage to congratulate Rik, to compliment Katrina and to pay their respects to Jackson's debut. Friends of his from the record label came in, laughing.

"I didn't know you were playing tonight Jackson!" Tony Flanders said. He was the A & R man for Dig It Records, and had come along to hear the new band.

"Well, fuck, Tony, what did you think?" Jackson asked.

"You were good. I never knew you played drums."

Rik laughed. "He never did either. I trained him good." Rik put his arm around Jackson's shoulder and gave him a hug. "For an American he knows timekeeping. None of this busy drumming, getting in the way of the soloist. I like that."

"For a European you're awfully opinionated," one of the musicians backstage said. "But you can play, I'll give you that. I'd like to sit in with you next set, show you an American player in action."

Rik nodded. "What do you play, my American musician?"

"Trumpet."

Katrina smiled for the first time since the set ended. "We're going to start with 'All Blues.' Can you play that?"

"Miss, I can play anything Miles ever wrote. The question isn't can I play it, but can he?" The trumpet player pointed at Rik and grinned.

"We'll see. Want a drink Jackson?"

"Mineral water please."

Rik went out of the dressing room with the crowd and to the bar. Katrina sat down next to Jackson and whispered in his ear, "Keep him under control Jack. He's really stoned tonight."

"I'll drive you guys home." Jackson offered.

"Thank you." Katrina paused a moment. "If his time starts to slip ... you'll support him?"

"Always Katrina." Jackson looked into the club and saw Henry Larkin standing by the door. He blinked twitched red red red his neck and looked again. Millie had just come in and was looking around for a table. "Oh Hell."

Katrina looked up. "What's wrong?"

"My ex-wife just walked in. Fuck shit bitch. I hope she doesn't see me."

Katrina grinned. "It will be hard for her not to. You're going to be on stage."

Jackson shook his head. "I haven't played since ... after the divorce. It will be weird to play jazz for her and him after all these years."

"Him?"

"My best friend. The man who broke up my marriage."

"Oh Jackson, I had no, what do they say, idea you had been married. Are you going to be all right?"

"Yeah. Don't tell Rik though. He'll probably make a scene."

"I know." Katrina kissed Jackson lightly on the cheek and walked out of the dressing room, shutting the door behind her. Inside the dressing room Jackson had a flurry of rapid neck tics, and began to grunt to himself. It was going to be a long evening.

FORTY SEVEN

The night that Jackson caught Millie and Henry in bed together was a bad one. Jackson had been at the record company late, as was usual those days, and had gone out with a friend to have a drink.

One drink led to two, than three, and by the time Jackson came home he was plastered. He sat out in the car twitching his neck and wondering why he did it. As he got out of the car he thought of Millie's soft skin and her warm eyes. He really had to spend more time with her, but somewhere in the last few months, since he had started his novel, he had gotten increasingly out of touch with her. He walked in, and noticed Henry's bass in the living room. That was odd. Sometimes he would come over and play for them but recently Jackson hadn't seen him. He headed to the bedroom. The door was locked.

"Millie?" Jackson said questioningly. He knew already, but had to hear to feel it.

From behind the door he heard voices, feverish and excited. Jackson sat down on the couch and nodded to himself. Well, it was bound to happen. Millie was an attractive woman, vital active sensual. But with Henry? Strong Henry, supportive Henry, the best friend of his childhood.

Millie came out, wrapped in a robe of soft silk. Her hair was down and she was slightly flushed still. "Jack ... "

"I know Millie. Why?"

"I was lonely. You had your book, your job. I had nothing, not even you." Millie began to cry and Jackson waited through her tears. She could turn them on without any trouble. "You won't hurt him?"

"Henry?" Jackson stood up and walked into the bedroom. "Henry, you motherfucker, come here."

By now Henry was dressed and sitting on the bed, ashen. "I'm sorry Jack ... " He began weakly.

"Take the bitch." Jackson said drunkenly. "I don't want to see either of you fuck again." His neck snapped hard, and he thought to himself, not now not here. But the tics were beyond his control in the emotion of the moment.

Henry left the house and Millie stood in the bedroom

138

with Jackson. "If I go Jack, I'm gone. I can't stand to see you drunk all the time waiting for the publisher to call. Do you want me to go?"

Jackson wondered how her going had become HIS decision. Well, make it then. "Go."

Millie leaned over him and kissed him on the lips softly.

"Goodbye Jack. I love you."

"Beat it."

Millie left the house and Jack heard Henry's car start. As it drove off he had an increasingly worse series of tics. He poured himself a scotch and turned on the television. "Oh good, *The Disenchanted*. Just what I need right now." Jackson settled down for a long night that didn't end even after the sun came up the next morning.

FORTY EIGHT

"You were great Jack." Millie said happily backstage. Henry was wisely still sitting at the bar from where they had watched the set. Millie was really beautiful tonight, Jackson thought. Her eyes shine - they float above the clouds like the stars at night. She hadn't looked that happy with him in, what, fifteen years?

"Thanks Millie. How are things?"

"I'm expecting." Millie held her stomach and Jackson had an incredible urge to punch her there. He held his arms tightly by his side until he could substitute the tic with something else.

"Congratulations. Henry's?" he asked viciously.

"No, as a matter of fact. We tried for years, I always thought it was you Jack, but it turns out I'm the one with fertility problems. So we had in vitro fertilization. Sperm bank withdrawal."

"Who'd you get? Helen Keller?"

"Jesus Jack, why are you so angry with me?" Millie had turned pale in the harsh light of the dressing room. Her eyes had turned from warm and inviting to cold and frightened. She sensed, for the first time in the twenty years she had known Jackson, the internal violence within him. It was not a sight she wanted to see. "We've been over for five years. Can't you move on?"

"I did move on and away and all of that. But you and that fucking Larkin keep on following me. Why the hell are you here tonight? What the fuck do you want from me? My money? I'm broke. My love? You killed it. My manhood? Well, it was never much, but you destroyed it. So leave me alone for once."

Jackson realized through the blur of red haze that they weren't alone. Rik and Katrina were standing in the doorway, appalled by his anger. Katrina came over to him and rubbed his neck. Rik looked at Millie for a long moment.

"Miss, please leave my friend."

Millie nodded and left, ashen. Jackson began to cry, totally spent. Katrina looked at Rik, and Rik left the dressing room, closing the door behind him. Katrina held Jackson for a long moment. Then she said softly, "we all need to go home. Would you like to spend the night with us?"

"I'd like that. I can sleep on the couch."

"Okay. Rik would like you with us tonight – he wants

to talk. When he's stoned he gets eloquent."

"Yeah, I used to get eloquent too. I also used to throw up a lot." Jackson watched Millie and Henry leaving the club as the door to the dressing room swung shut. He was alone again. Well, that's not true, he had the Van Beest's with him. But he felt alone as he always did when Millie left him. Five years. Shit, it seemed forever, it seemed like yesterday, it felt like NOW. When would he get over it? Would he? Jackson felt like he was in prison, solitary confinement with a red red red light for company. He thought of Millie's throat beneath his fingers. He tasted her warm lips in his mind and tried to remember kissing her. But the memory was dead, vanished in the years gone by, the tears having washed it away.

FORTY NINE

"You see Jack, all these women were bitches. To you they were glorious, romantic, beautiful. But they treated you like shit. You deserve better. When I think of the way this tramp cheated on you, abused your love ... "

"But I could have done better by her," Jackson started to say, still appalled at his earlier anger. It seemed that his self control had been eroded since he and Sara ended. First his rape of Maggie, now this verbal assault of Millie which could have turned physical if he hadn't stopped. Where was this new anger coming from, this hostility? Jackson didn't know and wasn't sure if he wanted to know. He just wanted it to end.

"Don't defend her." Rik said generously. "I think you want to feel guilty, to be the one at fault. You want to feel defective in this relationship. But she screwed around on you, remember that."

"But there are other crimes besides adultery. There's murder of love, accidental killing of passion and worse of all, boredom. I was guilty of all three."

Katrina came into the room, wearing a long flowing silk robe and holding two snifters of brandy. "It takes two to kill a relationship Jack. Here, you need this."

"No thanks. I shouldn't."

"God damn it Jack! Drink something, let go. Don't be so fucking controlled all the time." Rik thrust the snifter at Jackson, spilling a drop of brandy on the floor. It spread out like a bloodstain and Jackson winced. Red red red lying on the floor, red red red in my head and what's more ...

"Look Rik, if you want to drink, fine, go ahead. But leave me the fuck alone. I have tried real hard to stay sober the last three months. Don't fuck it up for me."

Rik started to respond, but at a harsh look from Katrina, stopped. "Look man, no problem. I can drink both of them."

Katrina laughed. "You'll have to help me tuck him in, Jack." Rik grinned and downed the first glass. He staggered to a chair and sat down heavily.

"We showed them, aye Jack? We showed them what jazz is, can be. Now we show them what a real movie can be. *Lucia*! God damn I love that bitch, your story is so ... so ... in here man." Rik patted his chest, burped and fell to the floor.

Katrina sighed. "He'll be out for days. Take his legs, I'll take his arms."

They carried Rik to the bedroom and Katrina covered him with a blanket. Jackson headed out of the room, somewhat embarrassed by his friend's stupor. It was too much like some of his own.

Katrina came out and sat down on the couch next to Jackson. He moved slightly away from her and she noticed. She moved to the other side giving him the space he seemed to need right now.

"I enjoyed tonight Jack. You could be a real player if you worked at it. I wish the triplets had stayed for the second set, when you and Rik traded eights ... "

"I liked your playing too Katrina. I wish Rik wouldn't push so hard."

"Why? Why do you care? He just likes to drink and snort. I wish he wouldn't take chances in clubs but at home?"

"I was an alcoholic, I am an alcoholic. It frightens me to see somebody that close to the edge all the time. I lived on that edge a long time and fell in a few months ago. It changes you, to face the edge, the hole in your life where the sun never reaches and death waits."

Katrina looked away. "I heard you tried to kill yourself. Is it true?"

Jackson closed his eyes, saw red red red, blinked five times and twitched his neck. "It's true that I put a knife to my wrists. Was it suicide? I can't say. I had wanted to die for a long time, since I was a child maybe, but I love my life too, even when the red gets in the way."

"Was it because of this woman, this Millie, that you tried to die?"

"Millie? I don't know. She was the first woman in my life, the only real relationship I have ever had. I gave her all my love but some things I couldn't give her. A baby, my full attention, me without the Tourette. All these things she wanted from me."

"What did you want?" Katrina leaned back and for a moment her breasts were outlined against her robe. Jackson looked away, then looked at her again. She smiled and sat upright again.

"What did I want? Oh, good sex, good money, artistic satisfaction. What did I get? Impotency most of the time from terror, bad money and debts from the divorce, fleeting moments when the writing felt good but now ashes ashes in my mouth. What do you want Katrina? To play bass in a jazz band, to be a mother, to be with Rik?"

144

"Those things are good. I like my triplets, they're good boys. I want to see them grow up happy. I love my music, I'd like to play some solo concerts like Miroslav or Dave Holland. Rik? Oh I do love him, but he's always going somewhere, doing something, never just sitting still. Like we are tonight."

"Katrina," Jackson began, then stopped. "I should go now."

"You said you would stay." She leaned forward and Jackson flushed. This didn't feel right.

"Rik is asleep."

"I'm awake. I played tonight too Jack, but the critics will write about Rik or you. Me? I'm just the bass player, you know, the pretty blonde on Rik's arm. I want more tonight. I want you."

"Well, you can't have me Katrina. I'm not much of a lover anyway."

Jackson said sadly but inside he felt proud that he could do the right thing for once.

"Hold me before you go? That's all."

"Okay."

Jackson held her in his arms and she squeezed him tight, her body pressing close to his. He stirred, and she moaned a little then kissed him on the lips lightly. She let go, and Jackson sighed.

"It would have been nice, Jack."

"It would have been wrong too."

"Yes, maybe. Good night."

FIFTY

"Just try and relax in the moment," Jillian said running her hand through Jackson's hair. They had reached the point in their therapy where Jillian wanted to try intercourse, to see if Jackson had learned enough about relaxing during sexual relations to enjoy all aspects of it. But inside Jackson curled a worm descending to his gut named impotency that was still alive despite the work between them.

"I told you about Katrina. How she wanted me."

"You told me you had refused her. Why?"

"Because Rik is my friend. Bitch puppies. Because I was more afraid of losing his friendship then hers."

Jillian laughed and ran her hand down Jackson arm to the light brown hair on his belly. He groaned and she smiled. "I think you're full of shit."

Jackson grinned. "I am. I was afraid I would be lousy in bed with her."

"A man with a perpetual erection isn't lousy. Just tiring."

"But a man with a limp dick is pathetic."

"Well, which shall it be today? Do you really want me, today, in this way." Jillian closed her hand around Jackson's penis and began to rub the shaft of it. He closed his eyes and twitched his neck once, seeing a warm pale red red red there.

"I'm ready. Oh yes." Jackson lied back as Jillian pulled a condom over his erection. Jackson rolled on top of her, his mouth seeking hers.

"No tongues Jack."

He laughed. "I'm fucking you and you're worried about ... don't stop, please."

He thrust into her again, lightly, and she moaned with him. Suddenly he closed his eyes as the room went white with light obliterating the red red red for a moment in a shrinking field of warmth. Jillian rocked with him as he came inside her. Sweat ran down his neck and pooled in the small of his back. He collapsed against her and laughed.

"So, that's what we've been working on. I like it."

"Good. I did too. You're not bad Jackson, for a beginner."

Jackson flashed on an image of Millie and shut his eyes, the pink inside them turning red red red. He twitched his neck and cried out "Damn it. I shouldn't be Touretting right now damn damn fuck shit ... "

Jillian sensed the emotion of the moment and held Jackson in her arms and legs, wrapping them around him like a blanket of human warmth. "Jack, dear, you can't stop the Tourette. Not ever. You can only hold it back for short moments of time while you're pleasuring yourself and your lover. But don't begrudge these moments, they make the silence, the lack of twitching, all the more special. You know Jack when I first met you I thought to myself, 'can I handle this? Will his noises his tics drive me away, make me hate him and by extension, myself?' But they didn't Jack. I got used to them. Millie got used to them. Sara was used to them. Everybody accepts your Tourette except you. Why Jack? Why can't you accept your imperfections as easily as you make apologies for Millie's? What is so wrong about being Jackson Evans?"

"I hurt." Jackson said simply. "I feel colors in my head, they burn so hot, they burn into my mind all the time. Red red red twitch your neck. Red red red shout 'fuck' or 'bitch'. Red red red demands and takes from me all the time and I have no more to give. Not anymore. I've written the best I could, loved the best I could, but it means nothing while the red red red is in me. Nothing means anything, has any value while I'm on fire with colors and touching the sound of burning flesh, tasting the heat and looking at the sound of fire in my soul. I can't love anymore because I'm death. I am red red red."

"But Jack, these are just more symptoms. They're you ... "

"God damn it. They're not me, they never will be! I let myself be the Tourette enemy inside me that drains my life of pleasure. I want to be real, be normal, be healthy."

"You are Jack. YOU ARE REAL - not sunken in fire but a living vital human being who can love and make love and enjoy it. Like you did just now. As you will again. With other women who can love you back fully."

"Until then, what? How do I hold on?"

"You just do Jack. That's all any of us can do, live in the moment. Experience the time you are in to its fullest and then move on to the next moment enjoying that too. You can't be focussed on the past - or in the future or even in the red red red that haunts your brain. It's not blood Jack! It's not death, it's life. It's you!"

Jackson looked at Jillian in wonderment, hearing her words and believing, and for a moment that lasted a long time the red red red was gone. He felt at peace here, in her arms, inside her. But when he withdrew, when he left, would it continue? To find out he moved away from her. She touched his back and her fingers left lines in the sweat there.

"Do I have to go now? It's been over two hours."

"Would you like to stay a little longer?"

Jackson thought of Millie and grinned at Jillian. "Can we do it again," he asked boyishly.

"Yes. Oh yes Jack. Can you? Can you live the moment and relax into it?"

"I can try." Jackson said simply.

"That's all any of us can do. Try. What a wonderful word."

"Thank you."

Jillian understood and touched Jackson's face. "It's gone, isn't it, right now you're not red red red?"

"I am red red red but I'm alive too."

Jillian laughed to herself. Jackson grinned and thought of it too. "You bitch. Say it."

"You're better red than dead."

Jackson groaned and held her tight. "Ready for a replay?"

"Go."

FIFTY ONE

It was a year later. Jackson entered the bookstore, his tan suit contrasting nicely with the brownish red beard he had grown in the past months. The bookstore owner saw him come in and walked up to him. "Are you ready, Mr. Evans?"

"Whenever you are." Jackson sat down in front of the pile of new copies of *The Honest Man* and softcovers of *Lucia*. He stayed at them and thought to himself, they are me, my words, my children. He thought of the screening of *Lucia* he had seen last night and how the audience had reacted to the new ending. Life was so much simpler in books, Jackson reflected. Rik thought the ending should leave you asking the question why? Why success, that bitch goddess we all worship? Why happiness, that devil who lures us along?

Why not, Jackson Evans thought to himself cheerfully. He looked at that first man in line and a frown crossed his face. He looked familiar.

"Sign this one to Linda." The man asked.

Jackson signed his name with a flourish. "Enjoy."

He looked beyond the man and saw a thin brunette

150

haired woman standing there. He blinked and stood up tensely. Jackson went over to her. "Hello Sara. Long time no see."

"You're probably wondering what I'm doing here. Why ... "

"No. I'm not wondering. It's your success too. I'm enjoying it."

Sara looked at Jackson closely. "You look happy Jack. Are you?"

"Yes. As much as I can be." He twitched his neck and held out his hand. "Dinner tonight? I know this great ... "

" ... Shish Kabob place?"

They laughed. Jackson went back to the pile of books and Sara watched him go, sad that despite his success he was still twitching, grunting and for all she knew still seeing the red red red. Maybe things would be better between them tonight.

"Do you think we could give it another shot, Jack," Sara said softly to him. Jackson pretended not to hear her but inside he felt a growing whiteness. Maybe things would be different this time. Did it really matter?

Jackson didn't know, didn't care, at the moment he was living in. He just was.

In the books they often end
without things resolved.
People are left hanging
Problems unsolved.

In the movies credits flash
And crowds cheer
And mermaids splash and rockets crash
And the end is near.

151

Echolalia

But to Jackson Evans and his life
He is content without a wife.
His books are produced
His love is seduced
His talents flourish and then
without a moan or a groan
He continues onward.

The writer inside
The tics outside
His books in the middle.

THE END

152